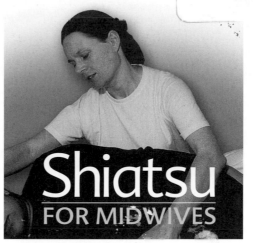

For Books for Midwives:

Senior Commissioning Editor: Mary Seager
Development Editor: Catharine Steers
Project Manager: Ailsa Laing
Design Direction: George Ajayi
Illustrator: Bruce Hogarth

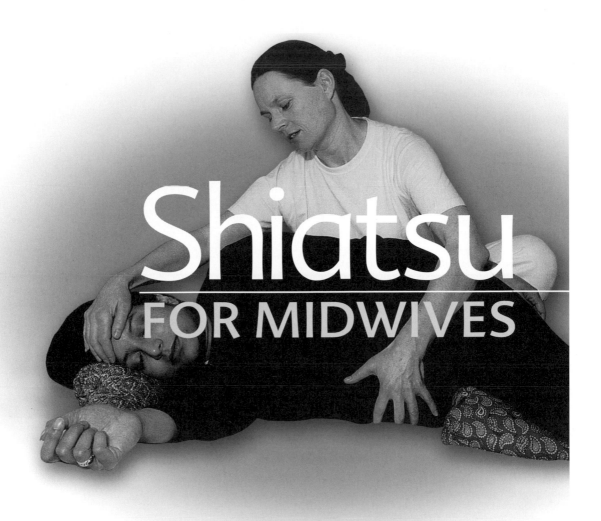

Shiatsu
FOR MIDWIVES

Suzanne Yates BA(Hons), DipHSEC, MRSS(T), Dip Therapeutic Massage (APNT), PGCE (PCET)

Director of Well Mother – Education for Maternity Care, Bristol, UK

With

Tricia Anderson BA(Hons), MSc, PGDip(THE), RM, SOM

Senior Lecturer in Midwifery, Institute for Health and Community Studies, Bournemouth University, UK

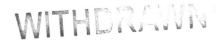

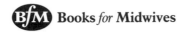 Books *for* Midwives

BOOKS FOR MIDWIVES
An imprint of Elsevier Science Limited

First published 2003

ISBN 0 7506 5523 2

British Library Cataloguing in Publication Data
A catalogue record for this book is available from the British Library

Library of Congress Cataloging in Publication Data
A catalog record for this book is available from the Library of Congress

Notice
Medical knowledge is constantly changing. Standard safety
precautions must be followed, but as new research and clinical
experience broaden our knowledge, changes in treatment and
drug therapy may become necessary or appropriate. Readers are
advised to check the most current product information provided
by the manufacturer of each drug to be administered to verify the
recommended dose, the method and duration of administration,
and contraindications. It is the responsibility of the practitioner,
relying on experience and knowledge of the patient, to determine
dosages and the best treatment for each individual patient.

Neither the publisher nor the author will be liable for any loss or
damage of any nature occasioned to or suffered by any person
acting or refraining to act as a result of reliance on the material
contained in this publication.

 your source for books,
journals and multimedia
in the health sciences
www.elsevierhealth.com

The
publisher's
policy is to use
**paper manufactured
from sustainable forests**

Printed in China

Contents

WITHDRAWN

Foreword

Having studied with Suzanne and incorporated some simple shiatsu techniques into my own midwifery practice as a result of her teaching, I was delighted to be asked to write the foreword to this timely book.

As we enter the 21st century childbirth in the UK – along with most Westernized societies – has reached a crisis point. Intervention rates are at an all-time high – our labour wards are increasingly full of expensive technology, with intravenous infusions, augmentation with artificial hormones and epidural anaesthesia commonplace. A woman having a normal, unmedicated birth is becoming an unusual event. The effects of this medicalized approach to the birth process can be seen in its results: Caesarean section rates of over 20%, instrumental delivery rates of over 15% and less than half of all 6-week-old babies receiving any breast milk. In many maternity units in the UK, a healthy primigravida has only a 1 in 2 chance of giving birth normally. She may enter the labour ward doors full of hopes and dreams, but too often leaves bruised, humiliated and shattered, nursing a wounded abdomen or perineum and a broken spirit.

Midwifery, the last bastion of normal birth, the traditional guardian of women's transition into motherhood, finds itself at a loss to know how to respond to this mass medicalization. While, on the one hand, midwives are the staunchest defenders of the normality of childbirth as a natural process in a woman's life-cycle, on the other hand they are busy learning to scrub in the operating theatre, site intravenous infusions and perform ventouse deliveries, as they adapt in order to survive in the medical world in which they find themselves. Midwifery has lost its way. But normal birth matters. It matters a lot. The work of Michel Odent and others has shown us how vital is the beautifully balanced hormonal process through which mother and baby pass in the course of a normal, spontaneous labour and birth. As they each experience their own peaks of oxytocin and endorphins, the baby is born alert, ready to feed and to attach to its mother, and the mother ecstatic and ready to love and bond with her new baby. The mother–infant relationship forms the elemental building block of all societies and cultures; if this relationship becomes contaminated with artificial hormones, painkillers, separation and pain, society will eventually suffer. Odent suggests we are seeing these effects already – in rising rates of ill health and social breakdown. It is this that makes the guardianship of normal birth – so hard in an increasingly technological world – such a precious task. No-one except midwives is likely to take on this role.

So where does shiatsu fit into all this? In order to try to reverse the trend, many midwives are searching for alternative ways to help women have healthy, fulfilling experiences of pregnancy and birth without recourse to the battery of pharmaceuticals on offer. The growing world of complementary therapies is an area to which many midwives are drawn, as are pregnant women who are attracted by the nurturing, holistic and personal approach exemplified by the best complementary therapists, which modern institutionalized maternity care so often sadly lacks. Midwives and women alike are increasingly frustrated with the inadequacy of the medical solution to many of the chronic symptoms of pregnancy, birth and the postnatal period – such as backache, insomnia, morning sickness, anxiety, slow labours, intolerably painful labours, heavy postpartum bleeding and problems with lactation. For these conditions, and many others like them, medicine has little to offer – and what it does have comes with a huge 'unwanted side effects' warning on the label.

Shiatsu has plenty to offer for these types of symptoms – which are, if you like, the bread and butter of a midwife's working day – and this is why this book will prove so useful. Shiatsu is based on the Eastern view of the body as an energy system encompassing the physical, the emotional and the spiritual aspects of ourselves. If all is in balance the person will be well; if any one aspect is 'out of balance', the result will be ill health and disease. A shiatsu treatment simply encourages the body to balance its own natural energy by gentle stimulation of its energy pathways, the meridians – the same pathways used in acupuncture. This approach matches perfectly the philosophy behind holistic midwifery; nurturing and caring for the interlinked triad of mind, body and spirit.

What is so fascinating to the midwife is how this theory, described in detail by Suzanne in Chapters 3 and 4, provides explanations for so many phenomena that midwives will have seen in their clinical practice, but for which Western medicine has no words. Have you seen women who sail through the first stage of labour, yet seem to falter when faced with the very different energetic demands of the second stage? Or women who seem to hold so much tension in their upper body that the cervical dilatation is slow and unproductive? Western obstetrics gives us no language to describe these kinds of phenomena, let alone to study or to resolve them. The Eastern model of the body provides us with an understanding of different types of energy, how each of us is more akin to one kind than another, and how energy gets blocked and can be released. Shiatsu, like acupuncture, is one method of doing this.

Suzanne is keen to point out that much of shiatsu is intuitive. If one is observant of the signals sent out by a pregnant or labouring woman's body, one's hands are naturally drawn to rub a tense shoulder, to squeeze an anxious hand or to stroke a tired forehead. We all know how soothing such a physical demonstration of caring can be. The age-old midwifery skills of touch and stroking are an intrinsic part of nurturing and cherishing: mother to child, midwife to labouring woman. Midwives around the world rub the lower backs of women in labour to ease the pressure of contractions. Shiatsu takes this simple healing modality of touch one stage further; within this book you will find suggestions of how to use what I believe are core midwifery skills of touch, gentle pressure and massage in a more systematic and focused way to help the mothers in your care. Women love it: I can testify to that!

There is more. As well as using shiatsu techniques to soothe and promote well-being, you will also find specific techniques here for many of the common problems of pregnancy, labour and early motherhood. From haemorrhoids to retained placentas, carpal tunnel syndrome to poor milk supply, the Eastern system of medicine explains many of these problems as symptomatic of blocked energy flows within the body, which simple shiatsu techniques can help release.

Midwives will be concerned about safety. While in many complementary therapies such as aromatherapy and herbalism there are genuine concerns about the safety of some treatments, especially in pregnancy, Suzanne Yates reassures us that shiatsu is about balancing the body's own natural energy: unlike many medical treatments, in shiatsu nothing is put in or taken out. As long as the person giving the shiatsu treatment does nothing that feels uncomfortable to her, and she stays responsive to feedback from the woman receiving the treatment, then she can do no harm.

The issue of following the new doctrine of evidence-based care is more complex. All midwives will be aware of the drive to rid ourselves of old, harmful practices which we inherited and which were never properly evaluated: shaves, enemas, routine episiotomies and continuous electronic fetal monitoring have all been shown to be harmful and have all rightly been consigned to the history books. Other 'routine' interventions are now coming under scrutiny and may gradually follow the same path. Learning from our mistakes, it is right and proper that all new practices should be fully evaluated before their widespread introduction. Suzanne Yates clearly tells us that shiatsu can do no harm, as long as certain commonsense guidelines are adhered to, thus fulfilling our primary directive of *'primum nocere'* (first do no harm): but can it do good?

The research base that exists to underpin shiatsu is discussed in detail in Chapter 2, but in summary, it must be acknowledged that there is only a limited amount relating to pregnancy and birth. Although shiatsu is based in an ancient tradition of touch and healing going back thousands of years, the modern-day shiatsu practitioner is a recent phenomenon. Shiatsu in the UK has only been formally established since 1981, and therefore the research base is in its infancy. But what little that exists is positive. There is some fairly robust evidence that suggests that the use of pressure on a particular shiatsu point on the wrist is effective in treating morning sickness: midwives may be familiar with recommending 'Seabands' for this condition. An initial practice audit in Bristol found that shiatsu was effective in inducing labour, and a full randomized controlled trial is currently being established. And importantly, the NHS systematic review on acupuncture, which uses exactly the same meridians and underlying principles as shiatsu, clearly demonstrates its efficacy.

So while the research base slowly accumulates, what are midwives to do? Midwives who begin to incorporate some basic shiatsu skills into their practice should certainly follow all the professional standards of obtaining consent from clients, documenting care given, auditing its effects and adapting their practice in the light of new research findings as they emerge. They can be confident they are doing no harm; and as what does exist is thousands of years of an empirical tradition and many anecdotal accounts of perceived effectiveness (read the fascinating case studies throughout this book), there is a high chance that they may be doing good. A shiatsu treatment certainly feels calming and pleasurable to the recipient. As so little of what midwives do to pregnant women feels good, and as we realize more and more the negative impact of stress on pregnancy outcome, then that fact alone supports midwives incorporating shiatsu techniques into their practice, while we wait for a more robust research base to evolve that studies the effectiveness of specific techniques.

Finally, a word on training. Midwives will be familiar with the Nursing and Midwifery Council's Code of Professional Conduct, which supports midwives to incorporate new skills into their practice, as long as they follow the principles laid out in the Code. Midwives are personally accountable for their own practice. They must not do anything they have not been trained to do, must ensure that the introduction of any therapy is always in the best interests and safety of their clients, and must ensure that they have had adequate and appropriate training. Now that the English National Board no longer exists to validate specific training courses, it is up to the individual professional midwife to assess whether her training and knowledge is adequate.

Suzanne is to be commended for her continuing hard work in trying to break down the barriers which often stand in the way of midwives applying a small range of selected complementary therapy techniques in maternity care, and thus prohibit women from receiving their benefits. Most midwives do not have the time or the money to spend 3 years or more on a full therapist training; what we need is specially designed, shortened but robust courses aimed at midwives, which are focused on the safe use of a limited range of treatments suitable for maternity care. Suzanne has devised such a course on applied shiatsu for midwives, which is focused on the needs of pregnancy, labour and the postnatal period and is sufficient to fulfil the NMC requirements. This is discussed in more depth in Chapter 2. Suzanne is the only shiatsu teacher in the UK to have specialized in maternity care work to the extent of making it the main focus of her work, and she has been working with midwives and pregnant women for the last 13 years. It is her accumulated knowledge and considerable experience in the maternity field that makes this book so unique.

I hope you enjoy this book. It takes midwives away from guarding technology and back to supporting mothers with their hands and their hearts.

The use of reassuring human touch has always been at the very heart of midwifery, giving women an anchor as they go through the storm of labour. In the modern midwifery whirl of science, academia and technology, the immense power of this fundamental midwifery skill has been overlooked. This book helps us rediscover it.

Tricia Anderson
Dorset, 2003

Preface

Who is this book for?

Although this book is primarily aimed at midwives, I hope that it will also be of interest to anyone wanting to know about the use of shiatsu in maternity care – including shiatsu practitioners, doulas and parents. Shiatsu was one of the main aspects of midwifery care in Japan for thousands of years, until the defeat of Japan in the Second World War and the subsequent medicalization of birth. Since then, only a few of the traditional midwives remain. I have been fortunate enough to have had access to some of their knowledge through a London-based midwife, Naoko Natsume, whose grandmother, Ikuyo Hosaka, was a samba (traditional midwife). Ikuyo was one of the first sambas to be trained in Western midwifery skills and she wrote about her work (in her self-published book 'My half-life record'). Naoko still uses some of her grandmother's techniques in her work as an independent midwife in the Japanese community in London.

Shiatsu in the West was initially taught mainly by Japanese male teachers, who had not accessed in detail the traditional wealth of knowledge on shiatsu and midwifery. Consequently, there is a dearth of good literature on the subject. There are many myths and much misinformation prevalent in the shiatsu community about shiatsu and maternity care. In my pursuit of a coherent model of shiatsu midwifery care, I have had the opportunity to share knowledge and skills with midwives and shiatsu practitioners worldwide; I hope that I have brought them together in a form which will be of use to all.

There are many traditions of shiatsu, from first-aid symptomatic point pressing lasting a few minutes, to a holistic therapy session lasting an hour. Some traditions, particularly those practised in Japan, are very vigorous physically and even painful to receive, while many Western practitioners have taken a more relaxing, energetic approach. What I am presenting in this book are examples of safe and effective work which can be done in a few minutes to several hours. It is possible, even in a short session, to work holistically rather than symptomatically and this is the approach I teach. I focus on relaxing, supporting techniques, as these are more appropriate in pregnancy, as well as more suited to being integrated into the practice of a midwife after short training.

Although to be a shiatsu practitioner requires a part-time training of 3 years, much of what is taught is not relevant to midwives wanting to use shiatsu for maternity care only. Shiatsu practitioners have to learn to work with the expressions of energy in all kinds of people with all kinds of illnesses. Shiatsu practitioners are required to study anatomy and physiology – which midwives know. Furthermore, shiatsu and maternity care is usually not taught to any great depth. A midwife can learn the most relevant points and meridians for pregnancy, birth and labour, and how to work in a way that carries an awareness of the whole movement of energy in the body, without doing a whole shiatsu course. This is why I developed a 6-day training course for midwives.

This book presents much of what I teach. It is about imparting basic instinctive skills in an accessible way. It will put across the key concepts and ideas behind shiatsu, but will also focus on some very practical skills which can, with appropriate training, become part of a midwife's core skills. The book is not intended to be a substitute for practical training. Practical skills need to be taught face-to-face so that corrections can be made and understanding confirmed. I do, however, believe that shiatsu is essentially an instinctive knowledge of touch and healing which we all have the potential to access. There were many healing touch-based traditions within our Western culture which, being oral traditions passed from mother to daughter, have been lost, especially during the witch burnings of the Middle Ages. I hope that by reading this book midwives will gain an understanding of what shiatsu is about, and that by following some of the basic principles they can rediscover skills, which they are probably using in some kind of rudimentary way, and be led to develop them.

How to use the book

The book is divided into four sections, each of which is relatively self-contained and focuses on a different aspect of shiatsu. You can go straight to the first section that interests you.

Section 1 is mainly focused on issues of relevance to midwives. Some aspects of it will be of interest to shiatsu practitioners, especially the sections on audit, research and the relationship between the shiatsu practitioner and midwife.

Section 2 is divided into two chapters. Midwives and those unfamiliar with shiatsu will need to read Chapter 3 (Key concepts) first before going on to Chapter 4, which is about the shiatsu view of pregnancy, birth and the postnatal period.

Shiatsu practitioners may well want to skip most of Chapter 3, although the sections on the development of the first meridians and the extraordinary vessels could be of interest.

Section 3 is divided into three parts. Again, midwives and parents will need to familiarize themselves with the 'basic principles' before going on to the specific chapters on shiatsu for labour, pregnancy and the postnatal period. Shiatsu practitioners will probably be most interested in the specific work first, but may find interesting ideas of how to present basic principles of shiatsu to their pregnant clients. I have written the 'conditions checklist' for midwives, so non-midwives will need to seek the advice of midwives or doctors before working with certain conditions – such as headaches, which may be an indication of pre-eclampsia.

Section 4 will be of interest to all as it contains ideas on how to adapt shiatsu exercises to pregnant clients. You can begin with this section – but if you want to understand the purpose of the exercises, you will need to refer back to the theory sections.

Throughout the book there are case studies to illustrate how shiatsu can be applied in midwifery practice. I have chosen to draw these mostly from the midwives who have attended my courses on shiatsu for midwives.

I have also chosen to use the pronoun 'she', rather than the more common 'he/she', as although there are male midwives, the majority are still women. I hope that male midwives and shiatsu practitioners will feel included despite the use of this term.

Suzanne Yates
Bristol, 2003

Acknowledgements

I would like to acknowledge the many different people who have taught me what I know about shiatsu and maternity care. Firstly, I can never thank enough my main shiatsu teacher Sonia Moriceau of the Healing Shiatsu Education Centre, who gave me such a solid foundation on which to build and develop my shiatsu knowledge. She not only taught me about shiatsu as a way of life, but gave me the opportunity to teach shiatsu – for which I am forever indebted to her. I would also like to thank Giovanni Maciocia and Shizuto Masunaga, who, although I have never met them personally, have inspired my work tremendously.

I have learnt so much from the many professional students I have had on my courses, massage therapists and shiatsu practitioners as well as midwives. Each student has taught me something new, and there are too many names to mention. I would especially like to thank the midwives who attended my courses and contributed directly to this book; Tricia Anderson, who went through the whole text twice and made me clarify my work as she did when she attended my course; and Naoko Natsume, who let me endlessly question her about her grandmother's work and helped me with Japanese references. I am also grateful to Carol Eames, Sheila Lawrence, Celina Domagala, Sister Hann, Julie Williams, Patti Saha, Alison Tilley, Karen Taylor, Liz Watts, Helen Parsons, Elaine Cockburn, Wai Choo McFarlane, Katharine Allen and Sarah Horan.

I would also like to thank Yae Nobuto, a Japanese shiatsu practitioner, and Andrea, an Austrian shiatsu practitioner, who gave birth in Japan and who provided useful information on shiatsu in Japan.

My thanks also to Zak, baby Kaylib, Wendy, Issie and Eva, who kindly posed for the photos in the book, and to Carolyn Hassan for the photography and advising me on how to present them.

Then there are the many hundreds of women I have been honoured to support during their pregnancies, births and the early months with their new babies. Without them, I could never have developed my work in the way I have.

And last, but certainly not least, I want to thank my family. Little did they realize how much they would inspire my work. My children, Rosa Lia and Bram Delaney, taught me, through direct experience, huge amounts about shiatsu during pregnancy and birth. They let me develop my shiatsu skills for babies and children and continue to demand that I work with them – which hasn't been easy while I've been teaching and writing this book. Also Chris, who learnt shiatsu for my births, and who continues to inspire and support me in developing my work. And finally to my mother, who gave birth to me at home and always inspired my belief in the positive aspects of birth with her message, 'the day I gave birth to you was one of the best days of my life'.

Glossary

Ampuku A Japanese form of massage pre-dating shiatsu, usually practised by blind people and still practised today.

Blood energy This is a form of energy – more than the Western concept of blood, it is not just blood in the blood vessels but also moves through the meridians.

Cun This is a Japanese/Chinese measurement for locating points on the body, representing 1 thumbwidth of the person you are working on.

Do-in A system of self-healing exercises.

Essence Known as Jing, it is the energy that underlies all organic life and is the source of organic change, controlling the reproductive function and fertility and supporting long-term growth and development.

Hara Approximately equivalent to the area of the abdomen, although it extends down to the pubic bone and up under the ribs.

Jitsu The condition of having too much energy in an area of the body.

Josanpu The Japanese nurse-trained midwife who came into being from 1947.

Ki The energy our body draws on from day to day.

Kyo The condition of having too little energy in an area of the body.

Makkho exercises A series of meridian stretching exercises, promoted by Shizuko Masunaga.

Meridian A pathway, either internal or external, through which energy flows in the body, sometimes known as a channel.

Midwife shiatsu practitioner A midwife who has also undergone the full professional training in shiatsu in his/her country.

Midwife trained in shiatsu skills A midwife who has done a short specific training in the use of aspects of shiatsu for midwifery practice.

Mother hand The hand that performs the Yin or supporting role when doing shiatsu.

Palming Using the palm of the working hand to work along a meridian.

Samba or sanba The traditional midwife in Japan prior to 1947. She would have undergone formal training in the Western midwifery approach and learnt shiatsu informally.

Sedation/dispersing Techniques for normalizing the energy of Jitsu areas, involving faster work and stretching.

Seiza The traditional Japanese way of sitting with the legs under the hips.

Shen Spirit, or human consciousness.

Shiatsu practitioner Someone who has undergone a full professional training in shiatsu (in the UK this is 3 years), but is not a midwife.

Shiatsushi The Japanese word for shiatsu practitioner.

Tao The whole.

Thumbing/thumb pressures Using the thumb of the working hand to work along a meridian.

Tonification Techniques for normalizing the energy of Kyo areas – involving slower, holding work.

Tsubo Acupoint.

Working hand The hand that performs the active or Yang role when doing shiatsu.

Yin Inward movement of energy represented by the shady side of the mountain, i.e. night.

Yang Outward movement of energy represented by the sunny side of the mountain, i.e. day.

Shiatsu for midwives

The aim of this section is to look at the main issues midwives need to consider when introducing shiatsu into their practice. It will cover professional issues specific to midwives, as well as issues of interest to shiatsu practitioners such as research, audit and the relationship between midwives and shiatsu practitioners.

1

What is shiatsu and what are its benefits in maternity care?

Introduction

Shiatsu is essentially a form of massage developed in Japan over thousands of years. Like acupuncture, its theory is based on the Eastern energetic view of the body. Vital energies such as 'Ki' and 'Essence' flow through the body along pathways known as meridians. The meridians pass through specific points – 'tsubos'. By balancing the energy of the meridians, a person's physical, emotional and spiritual energies are brought into greater harmony.

Shiatsu literally means 'shi' (finger) and 'atsu' (pressure) and it is characterized by techniques involving the use of perpendicular pressure. This pressure can be varied according to the needs of the client from barely touching the body to a deep penetrating pressure. It is a comfortable and deeply relaxing form of pressure and should not be experienced as painful. The practitioner is not limited to using pressure only at the tsubos used in acupuncture – any points on the body can be worked as indicated.

Pressure is not necessarily the only technique employed. Stretches can also be used to balance the energy in the meridians as well as massage-type strokes such as stroking and kneading. Touch may be combined with exercise and breathing. Midwives are often already doing things very similar to shiatsu as part of their care, like rubbing a mother's back or holding her hand. Shiatsu gives more focus and efficacy to these practices. There is no evidence of any side effects and much evidence of its effectiveness (for more information see Chapter 2).

Modern shiatsu developed in Japan in the 1950s and spread to the US and Europe from the 1970s; it has synthesized Western views of the body into its approach and includes work on the physical structures of the body such as muscle, bone and nerves. Modern shiatsu is constantly changing and growing – like the energy in the body to which it is responding and the different cultural context and traditions in which it is now practised. Many styles are practised worldwide. Some focus more on the Western, physical view of the body, others work with a more esoteric focus.

If you go to see a shiatsu practitioner, the session usually lasts for an hour and includes about 45 minutes of hands-on work. The rest of the time the practitioner will take a case history to make an initial diagnosis of the type of work required, and they will also allow time at the end for the client to rest or to show exercises or discuss other lifestyle issues. The client is usually fully clothed and lies on a cotton futon (mattress) on the floor, although with some styles of shiatsu, practitioners use a table and work directly on the skin with oil. Through pregnancy this format is followed, although the mother tends to lie more in the side position and, at the end of pregnancy, work may even be done in the all fours position to help encourage good fetal presentation.

Midwives can work in this kind of way if they have undergone the full shiatsu practitioner training, but there are many skills that can be integrated into their practice which may involve a few minutes of hands-on work during an ante or postnatal visit or hours of work during labour. This is very much how Ikuyo Hosaka used her shiatsu (for more information on her life and work see Chapter 3). In Section 3, I will highlight the techniques that she used and, indeed, the ones which I learnt from her via her grand-daughter Naoko Natsume.

The essential view that shiatsu embodies is of the body being a whole and the aim of the work is to balance energy flows, both to prevent and treat illness. In fact, in Japan, one traditional view of health was that the practitioner was paid when the client was well and not when they were sick. Shiatsu was seen as promoting a sense of well-being and thus a way of preventing illness from occurring. At the earliest level of a disharmony in the body, work can be done to prevent it from developing into something severe. For example, you can go to a shiatsu practitioner with mild abdominal pain which they can diagnose as a specific imbalance of energy and work accordingly to balance it. There doesn't have to be a tangible expression of that disharmony of energy. If left to the body's own devices, this energy imbalance may have eventually expressed itself as uterine bleeding, but by having shifted the blockages through shiatsu, it may be that no bleeding will develop. It is also possible to go and see the practitioner when there is bleeding and work may be done which slows or stops it.

The effectiveness of shiatsu depends on how stuck the energy pattern is and on the body's own ability to heal. Of course, if a woman is miscarrying a fetus which hasn't formed properly as a result of genetic defect, shiatsu can't magically make the fetus well. However, it can support the mother's body in the process of miscarriage. Shiatsu is often effective in preventing pre-eclampsia developing into eclampsia, but if the body has gone into eclampsic fits, then Western medication is the best choice of care. Since shiatsu is working with the body's own energy and not adding anything to it, it may be used effectively alongside conventional treatment. If shiatsu induction has failed and the woman is being induced with prostaglandins, it is still worth continuing to work with shiatsu points to help with the induction. If a woman has had an epidural, shiatsu may well help her use second-stage contractions effectively. In this sense, there are no absolute contraindications but extra care needs to be taken and close liaison with orthodox medicine is required in the more extreme situations of infections and inflammation, severe hypertension and pre-eclampsia, thrombosis (no direct work over the area) and cancer.

Shiatsu is not just about treating physical symptoms. The whole body is seen as one – the physical, emotional, spiritual entity. The medical model has tended to ignore the importance of the emotions of pregnancy. Emotions can become held in the body in ways that block the energy. The client doesn't have to express this to the practitioner. Indeed, if the emotion is held in the body, then it may well be that the client isn't even consciously aware of it. By shifting energy through shiatsu, the emotion can be released. This release does not necessarily have to be cathartic or dramatic. It may well be that the client simply feels more relaxed, more at ease, more at peace with themselves.

In the ideal world, a woman would have shiatsu before she conceives so that her energy is in the best possible state to begin pregnancy. She is then more likely to have an easier pregnancy, birth and postnatal recovery.

What style of shiatsu is being presented in this book?

I have developed my style of shiatsu in maternity care through my work with parents and midwives since 1989 when I conceived my daughter Rosa Lia. Recently qualified as a shiatsu practitioner, I was surprised by how little shiatsu was being used to support pregnant women. Shiatsu was still in its infancy as a therapy in the UK, and I was determined to use it as much as I could during my pregnancy. I had regular sessions from my main shiatsu teacher, Sonia Moriceau, and she and I taught my partner, Chris, some techniques he could use for pain relief during my labour. He used them so effectively, even helping to induce labour after my waters had broken, that I was able to use shiatsu as my only form of pain relief. More than that, it helped me to feel connected and positive about the whole process.

I was saddened by the negative culture around birth and wanted to promote a more positive attitude. Working with shiatsu was part of my vision behind creating Well Mother in 1990 to 'support the wisdom of parents and babies'. Chris and I set up 1-day workshops to teach other parents how to use shiatsu in labour. Initially, I was unsure how much others could use what Chris had done, as I was able to talk him through what I needed. However, I was amazed by how much even those fathers who were initially unsure or sceptical could take on the use of shiatsu. We have run regular workshops since 1990 and many parents have been able to rely on shiatsu alone for pain relief, even to induce labour, stimulate contractions, help reduce fetal distress,

aid downward descent of the baby and expel retained placentas. We still run these workshops. Parents feel more positive about the birth, and partners, whatever the outcome, feel glad that they have been able to be a supportive part of the process. Some partners have said 'I felt that I was giving birth myself'. When the mother uses only shiatsu during labour, she feels she has achieved something.

Case study 1.1   Parents' view of shiatsu use during labour – J and C on the birth of their baby

J: What I wanted more than anything was to help C in labour – to feel like I was giving something to her. Shiatsu gave me techniques such as sacral pressure and breathing together that were simple to learn and use. I felt part of my partner's labour, as if I had a definite role to play. Afterwards my partner said that even in the middle of it all she knew I was there and that made me very happy. The session beforehand with Suzanne was the first opportunity for us to express some of our hopes and fears together, and for the first time to really imagine what it would be like to be in labour together.

C: I found the shiatsu techniques connected us together during labour – something I really needed to feel. We used the sacral massage in the early stages – leaning over the bath during contractions. I was lucky in that my labour was quick and there were no complications. Nevertheless, it was still an overwhelming physical feeling and the shiatsu techniques enabled me to go through it without any other pain relief.

One midwife, who came on my parents' course when she was pregnant, was so inspired by the effectiveness of shiatsu, that she later signed up to do the full 3-year shiatsu practitioner training. She recently qualified as a practitioner and I include some of her case studies in the text.

Inspired by the success of imparting shiatsu knowledge to parents in 1 day, I determined to teach midwives these skills so that they could be used on a wider scale. I began by teaching short introductory sessions and demonstrations on complementary therapy days, and later, a day workshop at my local hospital. After some years I developed a 6-day course 'Shiatsu skills for midwives' which I have been teaching since 1998. I have taught the full course mainly in the UK, but have also taught some of the skills to midwives in Austria, France, Canada, Australia and the United States.

Unfortunately, today in Japan shiatsu in midwifery is a skill that is being lost. There are a few midwives who still use it, but most of the midwives in hospitals are focused on 'obstetric nursing'. Japan has become more and more fascinated by the ways of the West, as we in the West have become fascinated by the ways of the East. One of the latest fashions in Tokyo is 'British foot massage' – a school of reflexology was founded by a wealthy Japanese lady who studied in London. A Japanese woman on one of my courses commented that she has discovered more about shiatsu since she has been living in London than she knew in Japan. Western-style massage is more popular there than shiatsu. Although there are over 96 000 registered shiatsu practitioners in Japan, most of these have obtained their state certificate so they can work as a sports, beauty or aroma-massage therapist. The profession of 'shiatsushi' is not regarded that highly. Most pregnant women in Japan will not think of having shiatsu as part of their care.

The profession of shiatsu therapist, even in Japan, is a recent development. Before the 1950s, it was practised by blind people as a kind of massage – amna – as well as being commonly used as a home remedy. In Japan it is still widely used in the home. When someone feels ill, another family member will hold a point. They don't necessarily know the name of the point or the theory behind it. Magazines, the equivalent of 'Home and Garden', show which points to work and many gadgets to stimulate them are on sale in shops.

This home use differentiates shiatsu from many of the tools of modern maternity care. It is obvious that a woman cannot diagnose and prescribe for herself what drugs she may need to take. However, shiatsu is based on instinctive skills and tools – hands and body – which are accessible to everyone. Traditionally, in Japan, it was handed down within families as first-aid knowledge. Midwives would pass their knowledge down to each other without formal training. In our modern culture, where bodywork is no longer part of our instinct, we have to relearn how to connect with our bodies and with these skills. We could argue that the increasing use of technology in midwifery care which took place in the 20th century was a reflection of the greater role of technology in society as a whole, and changes in midwifery practice are simply reflecting this. Although we need to relearn what were once instinctive skills, this should not make us too anxious, in this litigation-driven society, about the safety aspects of using shiatsu. The body gives immediate feedback and no harm can be done if certain simple commonsense guidelines are adhered to.

The benefits of shiatsu in maternity care

Shiatsu can help to alleviate most of the common ailments of pregnancy, including morning sickness, carpal tunnel syndrome, back and neckache. It can help the mother to bond with her baby in the womb as there are techniques that include working directly through the womb and connecting with the baby's body. Some of these techniques include the use of light but firm pressure, appropriate to the baby's stage of development, and can be taught to the mother to use herself, or to the father, friends or family. Emotionally, it can help the mother become more aware of and in tune with her needs. In this sense, it can be a good preparation for the journey of motherhood and for the major transition of birth, both for the mother and father.

In labour, the fear of the unknown can be worked with. As all midwives know, unprocessed emotions can block the process of labour. Shiatsu can help a woman feel more connected with the intense emotions labour brings up and support her to let them work through her body. Pressure can be combined with stroking and breathing to provide effective pain relief in both the first and second stages of labour. There are some points that can be used to induce labour. Many midwives have successfully used these points and carried out practice audits which demonstrate their effectiveness. These same induction points can be used during labour to strengthen contractions and help with the descent of the baby. Some of them are also useful for expelling retained placentas. The baby can continue to be included in the work, which has the effect of calming the baby as well as the mother, and therefore reducing fetal distress.

Postnatally, work can be done with the mother to support her in establishing breastfeeding – both to help with the flow of milk as well as the quality of milk production. Shiatsu work is extremely useful for preventing and treating postnatal depression.

The mother and father can be shown how to use shiatsu on their baby which helps strengthen their family bond. Work with babies lasts for less time – often between 5 and 25 minutes depending on their mood – and can help them feel more connected with the big changes and adaptations they are going through. It can be done through the clothes, but is often done directly on the skin to help stimulate the immune system more directly. The stretches used in shiatsu are helpful for promoting the baby's physical development by facilitating the movements that the baby is exploring at different stages. With sick babies in neonatal units, shiatsu can be adapted to include extremely light pressure, even off-the-body work when too much body stimulation can be detrimental.

Summary of the benefits of the use of shiatsu

Benefits for the mother and partner:

- more likely to tune into her pregnancy – and therefore look after herself, pace herself, prepare for labour
- can deal with the 'complaints' of pregnancy, both major and minor
- more in touch with baby
- more able to trust in birth – that she can do it
- helps mother to cope with pain
- helps promote an easier postnatal recovery
- more likely to have a normal labour
- can promote a positive relationship with her partner, who can be more involved in pregnancy, labour and the postnatal period
- promotes long-term health.

Benefits for baby:

- helps baby to get in a good position for labour (optimal fetal position)

- more settled and at ease postnatally
- less likely to get distressed in labour
- natural support for many childhood diseases
- support baby's physical and emotional development
- more likely to have a close relationship with the parents.

Benefits for midwives:

- relaxing to do
- using hands-on skills
- working *with* the mother
- reduces the need to use medical interventions.

Benefits for the unit:

- cost effective as it doesn't cost anything beyond the costs of the original training and the midwives' time
- reduces the need for medical interventions, all of which cost money
- decreases the length of stay in hospital.

Long-term social benefits:

- promotes responsibility for health
- supports the long-term physical and emotional health of mother, father and baby
- supports the family unit.

Case study 1.2   Alison, community midwife, Worcester

I think that one of the things I have learnt most from using shiatsu, or been reminded of, is that midwifery is about being with women. It is about listening to their needs and really sharing their birth experience with them. Much of the intervention that takes place on delivery suites today is due to women being afraid because they are left alone – midwives are unable, due to staff shortages, to spend one-to-one time with labouring women. This in turn leads to more pain-relief requests as well as other interventions. The women I have worked with have demonstrated to me how important it is to be involved and in control, throughout their pregnancy and birth, in decision making for good postnatal outcomes to be achieved.

2

Professional issues

Introduction

At the beginning of the 21st century, there is an increased demand from women worldwide for all kinds of complementary therapies as part of their maternity care (Allaire et al 2000, BMA 1993, Department of Health 2000, Lloyd et al 1993, McCabe 2001, Tiran & Mack 1995). This raises many issues for midwives, not least what constitutes relevant training. One could argue that originally midwives were some of the first complementary therapy practitioners. Bridgit Lynch, in her moving keynote speech at the International Midwives Confe-rence in Vienna (Lynch 2002), referred to the traditional midwives of the Caribbean who inspired her in their approach to birth. These 'middis' told her that they were trained to work with their 'heart, hands and God'. The use of massage, herbs and intuition were the core skills of traditional mid-wives. In the drive to get midwifery accepted as a profession, much of this old knowledge has been devalued. Maybe now is the time to re-value some of these traditional skills, such as shiatsu. Complementary therapies have not been part of modern midwifery training but this is beginning to change. Many pre-registration courses offer complementary therapy modules (examples include Bournemouth University, University of the West of England, Greenwich University, Napier University), although most of these are more of a general introduction to complementary therapies rather than detailed training in the use of specific therapies.

Case study 2.1   Shiatsu as part of a complementary therapy module – Julie Williams, senior lecturer, midwifery, University of the West of England, Bristol

Shiatsu is one of the therapies included in our pre-registration midwifery module on alternative and complementary therapies. We have two sessions in which we introduce the basic concepts of shiatsu and encourage the students to practise some of the techniques on each other. The students usually enjoy doing this and most of them find it a relaxing experience. It also helps them to explore using touch on each other, particularly on the back, sacrum and the sacral grooves. These areas are good for using with women in labour, who often experience backache with their contractions and who could be offered back massage to help relieve this. We try to combine this with some other massage techniques so that they have something useful they are able to offer to women.

We also teach a few specific points such as Bladder 67, Gall Bladder 21, Large Intestine 4 and Heart Protector 6, which are relevant to midwifery and could be used for specific purposes without needing to have an extensive knowledge of shiatsu theory.

Having said this, the module is not intended to equip the students with sufficient knowledge to practise any of the therapies taught, but to offer an insight into them in relation to midwifery. If they wished to practise shiatsu or any of the other therapies, they would need to undertake further recognized training in order to do so.

This is highlighted in the Royal College of Midwives' (RCM) Position Paper (RCM 1999), first published in 1996, which emphasizes the midwife's professional responsibility towards his/her clients. These recommendations are timely and help to identify the parameters for implementing complementary therapies in midwifery. Previously, there was very little consensus on how, or even if, these should be used, with some hospital Trusts taking an enabling and positive approach, and others taking a much more cautious stance.

However, while it is good that some recommendations have been produced, the RCM paper advocates seeking out reputable courses which offer at least 500 hours of theory and the equivalent in practice. It may not always be possible to access such courses, and it is arguable whether midwives need to have this theoretical basis in order to practise just some aspects of shiatsu. Other professionals, e.g. vets, general practitioners (GPs) and physiotherapists, can offer complementary therapies on the basis of attending a short course in the appropriate therapy. Short courses in shiatsu *are* being run for midwives, and certainly some Trusts will accept this as evidence of sufficient training. It may be counter-productive to insist upon longer, more intensive courses if midwives cannot access these, so perhaps the RCM recommendations need to be more realistic.

It is also very obvious that clinical midwives are beginning to see the use of shiatsu, in particular, as a legitimate and effective way of providing care to women, whether in relation to optimizing fetal position, antenatal preparation, or for support and care in labour. Locally, there has been a small study carried out into the use of specific points for the induction of labour and a larger study is being planned. The prevailing attitude is very positive, with more midwives seeking out the necessary experience to develop skills in shiatsu and other therapies.

Perhaps it is appropriate to finish by stating that the last group of students who took this module found it a refreshing experience compared with the heavier, more theoretical modules that they were doing at the same time. If they are left with this impression, then perhaps they will be motivated to pursue some further training in shiatsu, massage, reflexology or the like once they are qualified. We certainly hope that we have aroused their interest in providing a more holistic and woman-centred approach to care.

Many registered midwives have undertaken their own complementary therapy training, either funded through their health authority or by themselves. A few midwives have trained in shiatsu, but not very many, as the full shiatsu training, similar to acupuncture and homoeopathy, is a 3-year part-time course. This has led to the wider use of therapies that are accessible through shorter training such as massage, aromatherapy and reflexology.

This raises the question of what is appropriate training, and whether midwives need to have done a full training in a therapy to be able to use certain aspects of that therapy in their practice. If midwives want to prescribe arnica for postnatal healing, do they need to have studied a 3-year homoeopathy course? If midwives want to support the mother in using lavender essential oil for

pain relief, do they need to be aromatherapists? Clearly, the answer must be 'no'. If a general practitioner (GP) can prescribe homoeopathic remedies after having undergone a short training, why can't a midwife do an appropriate short training course on the use of homoeopathy for midwifery? Denise Tiran states 'For midwives and others registered with the United Kingdom Central Council this (i.e. the need for appropriate and adequate education) does not necessarily mean that they must be fully qualified therapists, but that they must be able to justify their actions. It is … acceptable for a midwife to apply acupressure wristbands to the P6 wrist points to relieve nausea, so long as they have the relevant underpinning knowledge and understanding' (Tiran & Mack 1995). There are examples of this already in midwifery practice – midwives use listening skills without being fully trained counsellors or examine babies without being paediatricians.

Midwives already use many of the basic skills of shiatsu, such as touch and exercise, in some kind of way. If a midwife wants to encourage a posterior baby to turn and suggests the yoga cat position, it is accepted that the midwife does not have to be a trained yoga teacher to do this. If a midwife wants to use sacral pressure to help relieve the pain of contractions, she does not need to be a shiatsu or massage therapist as this is an accepted part of midwifery practice. Learning other sacral techniques and including the use of shiatsu points is simply an extension of the core practice and will probably improve the way midwives use sacral pressure.

As more and more women want to use some form of massage, including shiatsu for natural pain relief, one can argue that midwives need to respond to this impetus. Surely it is better for a midwife trained in midwifery shiatsu skills to teach women and their partners in antenatal classes how to use them effectively, than for women to pick up what they can from a book, or a friend who used shiatsu.

Professional and employment issues

Individual midwives need to define how much they want to integrate shiatsu into their practice. In all cases, the use of shiatsu must not be at the expense of normal midwifery responsibilities. For example, later on the book explains how to use shiatsu for induction – but of course all normal criteria as to whether induction is advised, apply. Most midwives will probably want to use shiatsu as an additional tool to help them in their work, and plenty of examples of midwives doing this are given throughout the book. They may want to use it as an option for dealing with some of the minor complaints of pregnancy; for teaching to parents as a self-help tool for labour; for using in labour; and for introducing parents to simple touch techniques for their babies. Other midwives may want it to form a bigger part of their practice and spend some of their time working in antenatal or postnatal clinics offering dedicated shiatsu sessions at specific times. A small number of midwives may want shiatsu to become the main focus of their work.

Case study 2.2   Sheila, community midwife, London

I have introduced shiatsu into midwifery practice with such good results that my Friday antenatal clinic has been filled with women whose babies are overdue so that I can combine the orthodox 'sweep' with some shiatsu techniques. This has been very successful. I use shiatsu with some labouring women too, where my contact with the woman is intense. Otherwise I am incredibly busy and overworked and it is basically more by chance than design that I am caring for a woman using shiatsu. I have demonstrated the theory and practice very basically for a group of midwives on a teaching and assessing course at Thames Valley University. With courage and confidence, I gave a talk and demonstration to a group of midwives at the Chelsea and Westminster Hospital as well as contributing to a session at St Mary's Hospital.

Case study 2.3   Liz, community midwife, Southampton

I am based at the Princess Anne Hospital in Southampton and do a weekly antenatal clinic in a GP's surgery. I work mainly in the community but also work some shifts at the hospital. I use shiatsu quite a lot in my work as a midwife. Most women I see are in my antenatal clinic but I do not get much time to see them as most appointments they have with me are only 15 min long. I have had success in helping them to use shiatsu to ease minor disorders of pregnancy, such as nausea, carpal tunnel and backache. I teach them postural exercises such as the 'all fours' and leaning forwards, and do some quick work on the sacral points. They tell me when I have found the right spot. I also help with symphysis pubis discomfort by placing my hands over the symphysis and the lower back while asking the woman to breathe slowly while I apply pressure on the out-breath for a few breaths. This is very effective for pain relief in labour and several women have gone on to give birth quite quickly after I have used this technique. I show their partners how they can help.

I have used reflexology with the shiatsu points to help labour become established with several women. These women have been admitted to hospital for induction of labour and if I have time I will spend up to an hour with them. If they require Prostin induction I can work on their feet and lower leg points while they are being monitored following the medical induction. Some babies become quite active following the use of the induction points, as recorded on the cardiotocography. The women enjoy the attention and find the shiatsu relaxing.

In all countries the midwife needs to pay attention to any guidelines relating to midwifery practice, in particular those relating to the integration of new skills in general or complementary therapies where specific guidelines apply. In the

UK, the main criterion from the Nursing and Midwifery Council (NMC) (Nursing and Midwifery Council 2002) is that midwives 'must ensure that the use of complementary or alternative therapies is safe and in the interests of patients and clients. This must be discussed with the team as part of the therapeutic process and the patient or client must consent to their use'. In the US midwives should refer to the American College of Nurse Midwives guidelines (American College of Nurse Midwives 1993).

In the UK, the United Kingdom Central Council (UKCC) Midwives' Rules and Code of Practice (United Kingdom Central Council 1998) reminds midwives that the needs of the mother and baby must be the primary focus of their practice. It goes on to state 'Some practising midwives, having gained a qualification in a complementary therapy, want to apply their additional knowledge and skill in their practice. It is essential that practice in these respects, as in all others, is based upon sound principles and upon all available knowledge and skill. You must obtain consent from the mother to the use of such therapies. Your professional accountability applies in the use of such therapies as in any other area of practice'.

It may be helpful to remember that shiatsu, unlike the other commonly used complementary therapies (homoeopathy, aromatherapy and herbalism), does *not* involve introducing any foreign substance into the body and therefore does not need to be considered in the same light, with the very real concerns about safety of the administration of medicines. The Code of Practice makes this distinction by having a separate section on the administration of homoeopathic and herbal substances. Shiatsu, on the other hand, is an applied bodywork and massage technique, which has negligible unwanted side effects (as discussed in more detail on p. 22 and 180).

It is clear from the UKCC guidance that as long as a midwife, who is always individually accountable for her practice, ensures that a sound rationale can be provided for any treatment that is given, based upon the best available knowledge and skill surrounding the use of shiatsu in maternity care, then she is abiding by the Code of Practice.

The UKCC does not prescribe what constitutes 'a qualification', leaving it up to the individual

midwife, in discussion with the supervisor of midwives, to assess whether the training course that has been undertaken is sufficient preparation to utilize a limited range of applied shiatsu techniques using 'sound principles and upon all available knowledge and skill'. The Nurses Board of Victoria, Australia (1999) refers to different competence ranges, 'from a basic level, with guidance from an experienced practitioner, to an advanced level practitioner', and the midwives can 'use complementary therapies according to their level of knowledge and competence'.

In the UK, the Code of Professional Conduct issued by the NMC in 2002 clearly lays the responsibility of assessing one's competence to practise new skills acquired following registration in the hands of the individual professional. Now the English National Board no longer validates individual programmes of study, it is up to individual midwives to assess whether the course they have followed has given them sufficient theoretical knowledge and practical experience.

Sue Way, Midwifery Education Officer at the NMC, explains 'It is important to emphasize that each registrant is accountable for ensuring they have the knowledge, skills and competence to carry out the care they are engaged in. The position in relation to midwifery practice is set out in the Code of Professional Conduct and Midwives' Rules and Code of Practice. The NMC believes that these two documents together provide key principles to underpin the scope of midwifery practice' [personal communication].

In relation to extending the scope of professional practice to include skills such as shiatsu, Sue goes on to say that 'more generally, midwives should be able to give evidence to their manager that the course provides them with the knowledge, skills and competence to support extending their scope of practice'.

If midwives want to be potentially able to work in all situations, then they will want to do the full shiatsu practitioner training. If, on the other hand, they want to use shiatsu as a small part of their work, then it is not necessary to do the full training. Provided that only the specific shiatsu skills are used for which training has been given, then shorter courses will satisfy the NMC criteria.

There are precedents for this differentiation – many doctors use homoeopathy in their general practice after having undergone short courses, but they are not homoeopaths. Similarly, vets and physiotherapists use acupuncture in their practice after having undergone a short training, without having completed the 3-year acupuncture training.

Midwives at John Radcliffe Hospital, Oxford, use a limited list of aromatherapy oils without having undergone a full aromatherapy training (Burns et al 2000). Managers and supervisors have accepted Suzanne's 6-day course on shiatsu skills for midwives as adequate training for midwives to use shiatsu in their work.

Midwives need to have the appropriate theoretical underpinning and understanding, and be aware of what they have been trained to use and the limits of their understanding. They need to know what to do if they are unsure, and to have mechanisms in place, such as contact with shiatsu practitioners or peers, to have support in these situations. As long as they are aware of what they are doing, this is 'acceptable practice'.

Developing a protocol

A protocol needs to be developed for each unit/ Trust where midwives intend to practise shiatsu in any form. A protocol needs to include clarification on issues including:

- a definition of shiatsu
- training criteria
- eligibility for women's inclusion
- informed choice/consent
- record keeping and audit
- evaluation form
- professional issues
- employment issues
- insurance
- role of lay shiatsu practitioner
- standards for audit.

A definition of shiatsu

This needs to include information about how shiatsu is going to be used. It can include a summary of its benefits in maternity care and any cautions/ contraindications.

Training criteria

This would indicate the type of training required and what it enables the midwife to do. If it is a short training course, then midwives must only practise within the limits of what they have been taught. They must submit copies of certificates to the head of midwifery services.

Eligibility for women's inclusion

Shiatsu can be used in a wide variety of situations, from alleviating anxiety during pregnancy to expediting delivery of the placenta. It is therefore not appropriate to have a list of inclusion criteria. However, midwives must be mindful of their professional responsibility to liaise with the full multidisciplinary team and to refer to an appropriate professional when a deviation from the norm is detected as outlined in the NMC's Midwives' Rules or the relevant rules in their country. They should also ensure that using shiatsu techniques should not take precedence over their essential midwifery skills, knowledge and training.

Informed choice/consent

Informed consent remains a fundamental tenet of all professional practice. The NMC states that 'you must ensure that the use of complementary or alternative therapies is safe and in the interests of patients and clients. This must be discussed with the team as part of the therapeutic process and the patient or client must consent to their use' (NMC 2002). Informed consent must be given by the mother after shiatsu has been clearly explained and its use documented in her notes. An information leaflet can be provided for clients which explains the principles of shiatsu and its application in maternity care. This leaflet could also include a space for giving informed consent (see Appendix 1, pp. 174–175). A copy of this could be kept in the case notes.

Record keeping and audit

Provision needs to be made for keeping a record of the use of shiatsu in individual care. Clients need to be aware of this and give consent for records to be used retrospectively and for research purposes.

Evaluation form

This can include space for:

- how shiatsu affected the care from the midwife's perspective
- how the woman experienced the shiatsu.

Criteria such as effectiveness and comfort can be measured.

Professional issues

All midwives must give full attention to the guidelines of the professional regulating body in their country. These will include the code of professional conduct, the code of ethics and other relevant guidelines. In the UK this is the NMC's Code of Professional Conduct and the Midwives' Rules and Code of Practice (NMC 2002).

Employment issues

All midwives who are appropriately trained and wish to integrate shiatsu into their routine midwifery practice must pay attention to the contract they have with their employer and any relevant policies where they work.

In the UK this involves contacting the head of midwifery services to discuss and agree on the parameters in which to practise. The head of midwifery can then draw up a list of names of the midwives and disseminate this list amongst staff and clients. The midwives also need to discuss their plans, along with their arrangements for appropriate support, practice, audit and ongoing education with their supervisor of midwives. They need to be able to provide evidence of appropriate preparation and education and provide a copy of their certificate or diploma to the head of midwifery services and their supervisor.

Insurance

Midwives need to check that they are adequately insured. In the UK, as long as the head of midwifery has agreed that the midwife can use shiatsu as part of her NHS midwifery practice, appropriately trained midwives who are employed by the NHS will be covered by the NHS vicarious liability scheme. Midwives are advised to discuss this with their head of midwifery. The RCM also provides medical malpractice insurance cover for full members who work for an employer who assumes vicarious liability for care given on its behalf. This includes midwifery duties that an individual is competent to undertake (including complementary therapies) where an individual is undertaking such care within the overall sphere of NHS midwifery practice with the knowledge and approval of the management and supervisor (RCM 1999).

If midwives want to practise independently from their employer, they will need to organize their own insurance. The Shiatsu Society provides insurance for fully qualified practitioners. Other organizations such as the British Complementary Medicine Association (BCMA) may provide insurance for some short courses.

Role of lay shiatsu practitioner

A client may choose to bring her own shiatsu practitioner into the maternity unit, and she should agree this in advance with the head of midwifery.

If the hospital wishes to contract in a lay shiatsu practitioner, the practitioner will be required to show evidence of professional insurance cover and training in maternity aspects of their therapy.

Standards for shiatsu strategies in maternity care

Clinical governance clearly puts the responsibility for the standard of clinical practice in the hands of the practitioner. In initiating any new approach to care, clearly auditable standards need to be set by the clinicians involved, in discussion with management and the full maternity care team. What follows are some suggestions for standards which should be audited annually. It may be appropriate for a named supervisor of midwives who has a special interest in complementary therapies to take responsibility for supporting midwives who are using them in their practice.

Standard no. 1

Midwives need to demonstrate a practical understanding, backed up by theory, of the use of shiatsu in specific situations including antenatal care, labour, postnatal care and care for the baby. This includes the use of exercise and posture.

Audit criteria:

- Midwives record the mother's consent in the notes.
- Midwives record their use of shiatsu in the mother's notes – including what they do and what is the effect.
- Midwives receive annual updates on their practical skills.
- Midwives review their practice regularly with other midwives trained in shiatsu skills, midwife shiatsu practitioners and shiatsu practitioners.

Case study 2.4   Setting up a shiatsu service in the Borders General Hospital, Scotland – Sarah, hospital midwife

Aims
To raise awareness of the availability of shiatsu in the Borders General Maternity Unit both to pregnant women and to fellow midwives.

How
Information leaflets are displayed in the antenatal and postnatal wards, antenatal clinic and peripheral clinics. The availability of shiatsu is discussed in parent-craft classes.

Contact numbers for relevant staff are listed on an information sheet for women to contact directly or to leave a message.

There is no set appointment time for shiatsu; it is carried out in midwives' rostered duty time, and mainly given on an ad hoc basis.

To raise staff awareness there is a resource folder in the labour ward for staff to dip into as they wish; staff are encouraged to use makkho ho exercises for self-development/relaxation.

Currently, shiatsu treatment is documented in the patient notes, and midwives keep a personal record.

To develop
Talks to staff to inform them further of the uses of shiatsu and to raise awareness.

A database of patients and treatment given, follow-up, feedback on treatment.

Record card.

Depending on the level of uptake of therapy, the possibility of using clinic time for prearranged appointments.

Standard no. 2

Midwives need to consider issues relevant to the integration of shiatsu into midwifery practice.

Audit criteria:

- Midwives annually review their protocols for guidelines on the use of shiatsu.
- Policies are updated annually in the light of new research/experience.
- An annual client satisfaction survey is undertaken and the service reviewed in the light of its findings.

Shiatsu training and regulation

In each country where shiatsu training is offered there is a national or state regulating body (see Appendix 2). The national regulating body for shiatsu in the UK is the Shiatsu Society and they hold a register of the schools in the UK who provide training that meets their required standards. In each country the regulations governing the use of shiatsu are different and you need to check the law in your country. In England and Wales regulation is voluntary, so in theory anyone can set themselves up as a shiatsu practitioner, as long as they do nothing against the law. In practice this doesn't often happen, but it is still advisable to check the qualifications of shiatsu practitioners.

If a midwife wants to work as a shiatsu practitioner, then the training in the UK is a 3-year part-time course. This is usually with a shiatsu school, although there are now some universities that offer the full shiatsu training as part of a BA degree level course in complementary and holistic therapies (e.g. University of Derby). The course covers all aspects of shiatsu – learning all the meridians, both the theory and how to work them, as well as anatomy and physiology and some basic counselling and practice management skills. Different schools may emphasize different styles. Some focus more on traditional Chinese medicine, including skills such as tongue and pulse diagnosis, cupping, moxibustion, the use of herbs and diet. Others focus more on the meditation, self-healing and exercise aspects of shiatsu. Most schools offer introductory weekends and so it is worth attending one of these to see which style of shiatsu you prefer.

It is worth checking the qualifications of anyone who will be teaching and ensure that they are registered as a teacher with the Shiatsu Society. The Shiatsu Society publish a booklet with a full list of teachers and schools in the UK, available on application to them or via the website (www.shiatsu.org).

The 3-year course does not tend to cover maternity care in much depth. Some schools offer an introductory day or a weekend on shiatsu and maternity care in the third year, others do not even offer that. When choosing a school, you may want to ask what they teach about pregnancy, birth and postnatal care. I constantly meet shiatsu practitioners who say that they have developed a fear of working with pregnant women because they only know what not to do, rather than what they can do. Many don't have a real understanding of the antenatal, intrapartum and postnatal periods. I teach introductory days and weekends for shiatsu schools and have created a postgraduate course of 14 days spread over a year to teach shiatsu practitioners more about maternity care. As far as I know, this is the most in-depth maternity-work course for shiatsu practitioners and I teach it worldwide. Even midwives who have studied the full course may still want to access more specific maternity training in shiatsu when they have qualified.

Many shiatsu schools offer short courses or foundation courses which teach the basic principles but not the use of the more complex diagnostic skills. Some schools provide a licence to practise and insurance after this training. Although this covers basic skills, it does not usually include specific training on the use of shiatsu in maternity; midwives need to be very careful what they use from these shorter training courses in their work and will need to follow-up the training with some specific maternity training.

Midwives wanting to use specific shiatsu skills in their work will need to attend a specialist short course on shiatsu and maternity care. At present, I am the only registered teacher in the UK to offer such a course, but I hope to expand this and am working at supporting shiatsu teachers worldwide to provide this type of course. This course has been recognized by several Trusts as evidence of appropriate training. It has been accredited in the US for continuing education and I am currently in negotiation with accrediting bodies in the UK.

Some midwives may find that their employer will fund some or all of their training for the shorter courses. There are also scholarship schemes supported by the Royal College of Midwives and local grant-awarding Trusts that midwives can access.

Continuing Professional Development in shiatsu

Peer support – the relationship between a shiatsu practitioner (midwife or non-midwife) and a midwife trained in shiatsu skills

If a midwife decides to take one of the shorter courses, then she will need to make sure that links are made with a local shiatsu practitioner who specializes in maternity work and who may or may not be another midwife, to establish ongoing support and supervision. In forming this relationship, the midwife will want to check the training the practitioner has undergone in maternity work, and their insurance and registration situation. The midwife may want to ask questions about how much the shiatsu practitioner has worked with pregnant women, their experience of shiatsu in labour, the early postnatal period and with babies. In deciding who is a suitable practitioner to work with, it is often a good idea for the midwife to experience some shiatsu from several practitioners.

This can be a beneficial relationship not only for the midwife, but also for the shiatsu practitioner, who can learn from how the midwife is using shiatsu in her work. For most shiatsu practitioners, maternity work is usually only a small part of their work and the midwife may quickly build up more knowledge than them in the maternity field.

One model for this kind of relationship is the mentoring or supervision model. The midwife and practitioner may want to meet regularly to discuss issues which are relevant or they may meet to discuss specific cases. They may even decide to set up a support group, with one practitioner offering supervision to several midwives. Another model is the peer review and support model.

Networking

Midwives can develop their knowledge of shiatsu by networking with midwives in other areas who are using shiatsu. These opportunities can be used to support research projects.

Reflective diary

As in all areas of practice, midwives need to make sure that issues and themes of relevance to shiatsu are entered in their reflective diary.

Ongoing training

All midwives and shiatsu practitioners need to show evidence that they are continuing to update their skills by regularly attending relevant study days. For a midwife trained in shiatsu skills, this may involve extending her knowledge of shiatsu by attending the first year, or more, of the 3-year shiatsu course.

Reading, audit and research

Midwives need to continue to study on their own and to engage in audit and research opportunities to do this.

Research

In these days of research/evidence-based practice, it is important to consider the research base on shiatsu in order to be able to justify one's actions. It is also important to realize that shiatsu is a therapy that has been around in essence for thousands of years and there is a lot of evidence as to its safety and efficacy which hasn't necessarily been formalized into a randomized control trial.

There is not a great deal of research specifically on shiatsu; a lot of the research mentioned in this chapter relates more to acupuncture for which there is a much larger research base. The main reason for this is probably because shiatsu in the West (UK, Australia, North America, Europe) is a relatively new therapy; it tends to attract people who want to work in an intuitive, hands-on way and its therapeutic use in Japan is limited. Shiatsu

is increasing in popularity worldwide but is still less widely used than acupuncture and massage, which became established first. In the UK, it has only been used on a wide scale since the 1990s. In 2002 there were 1672 registered practitioners, a number which is increasing year by year. In many states of the US, to practise shiatsu you also have to be registered as a massage therapist and so shiatsu is often only taught as part of massage training. In Canada, following lobbying for shiatsu as an independent profession, this is not the case. Shiatsu in Japan has unfortunately declined since the Second World War and it no longer has a strong foundation in its land of origin. There are some shiatsu schools in Japan, but most of the respected teachers, either Japanese or non-Japanese, live outside Japan. This means that little research is available from Japan.

Acupuncture became established worldwide before shiatsu and so there are greater numbers of practitioners. Acupuncture has also retained a strong base in its homeland of China, where its traditions were valued and researched greatly during the Cultural Revolution in the 1950s and 1960s. Although much of that research was not carried out to particularly high standards, in China today there are many universities and colleges offering good courses in all aspects of Chinese medicine, from acupuncture to herbs to manual bodywork, and which are carrying out better designed research studies.

In looking at the research base on shiatsu, I argue that we can consider studies on acupuncture and massage as well as the limited studies specifically on shiatsu. Shiatsu is essentially based on the same system as acupuncture – if acupuncture works and is safe, then so is shiatsu in terms of its therapeutic model. Indeed, many of the acupuncture studies have been done using acupressure: stimulating points with pressure rather than needles, which is a form of shiatsu, and some studies combine shiatsu and acupressure (Ballegaard et al 1996). Shiatsu could be considered as less invasive and therefore it could be argued that it is potentially safer than acupuncture. Some studies on massage will be considered because shiatsu uses techniques which are forms of massage.

Research into both shiatsu and acupuncture poses problems for the modern researcher. Given the fact that there is not one 'cure' or 'technique' for a particular illness (as shiatsu and acupuncture are about balancing the individual energies of a person), they are more difficult to research using a randomized control trial. In order to satisfy measurable criteria, research can become oversimplistic. It is amazing that research has shown benefits when it is looking at the use of a specific point such as HP-6 for nausea. One would expect that only a certain number of people would respond positively to such a point. For others, different points and work would be more effective. Bensoussan (1991) explores in detail the issues facing researchers in the field of acupuncture and the importance of understanding how the system works so that they can frame the right question and design the study accordingly.

Many studies that have been done have been criticized for not having used appropriate methods of research. The Cochrane Reviews on some of the acupuncture and acupressure studies in pregnancy recognize none of the studies because they do not fit their criteria. The National Health Service (NHS) Centre for Reviews produced a systematic review of acupuncture studies by reviewers from the complementary field of the Cochrane Collaboration; it concluded that many of the trials are of poor quality, providing insufficient evidence to guide clinical developments (NHS Centre for Reviews 2001). The review identified a need for better designed studies, although it did conclude that there is evidence of acupuncture's effectiveness for postoperative nausea and vomiting in adults, chemotherapy-related nausea and vomiting, and postoperative dental pain, and that it is relatively safe in the hands of suitably qualified practitioners, with serious adverse effects being extremely rare.

The problem with many of the studies is that they are small and poorly designed, the data are subjective and there is not a true placebo. More recent studies are beginning to address the limitations of previous studies, but it is important not to negate the volume of research which does exist, as it indicates many useful areas for more rigorous research, and equally importantly it has never come across any side effects.

In research, it is difficult to isolate the placebo effect. To atttempt to isolate it, the control group needs to have some kind of touch intervention which is non-shiatsu specific. This way it is possible to research how much difference shiatsu makes when compared with unfocused touch and support. A second control group may then be needed to act as the baseline for no intervention at all. Sometimes people argue that shiatsu works because of the time and physical contact and that it could be solely this which is important. This is not necessarily an argument against shiatsu in this culture of increasing reliance on machines and technology. Just the close contact of one person to another can be a big part of the therapeutic effect of shiatsu – and who is to argue that this is not a valid reason for using it. There has been research on the role of the doula in labour which validates the importance of this (Hodnett 2002).

There are certain aspects of shiatsu that can be researched quantitatively. I am involved with developing a randomized controlled trial on the use of shiatsu for induction which will involve large numbers of women. The use of a selection of points for induction has been proposed and a way of working which will address individual needs.

There have been arguments put forward for more qualitatively designed studies – such as case study analysis or providing individual shiatsu for specific illnesses and researching its effects rather than a specific intervention. One such study was carried out in which 11 patients received shiatsu once a week for 5 weeks. Unstructured interviews were conducted to draw out information, and the study offers useful insights to help guide future research (Cheesman et al 2001). The drawback of this method is that by necessity it is difficult to research large groups of the population.

This raises another issue as to why there is not much research on shiatsu. Shiatsu is about hands-on work and does not generate a specific product which can be sold, other than the training of therapists. There is no money to be made by a multinational company which means that there is little money available from these companies to fund research. This is also one of its benefits – ultimately it is very cost effective as the only costs involved are relevant training and the hours of the caregivers.

There is a lot of scope for midwives to contribute to developing the research base on shiatsu.

By carrying out ongoing practice audit, they create the basis for guiding subsequent controlled research. Following the 'Shiatsu for midwives' course at St Michael's Hospital, Bristol, an audit was carried out on the use of shiatsu for post-term pregnancy. This involved a midwife in the post-dates clinic doing some shiatsu on women and then showing them how to use specific points and techniques on themselves. The audit showed that post-term women who used shiatsu were more likely to labour spontaneously than those who did not. Of the women who had used shiatsu, 66% (42/66) went into spontaneous labour compared with 36% (26/77) of women who did not use shiatsu. The 'shiatsu group' had a significantly lower rate of inductions and slightly fewer Caesarean sections and instrumental deliveries. These preliminary findings suggest that savings could be made both in terms of the cost of inductions and time spent in hospital postnatally. Now a randomized control trial into the use of shiatsu for induction of labour is being explored and has already gained ethics committee approval.

Summary of the research base on shiatsu, acupressure, acupuncture and massage to support the use of shiatsu in maternity care

The research base on how shiatsu works is described in Section 2. What follows is a discussion of the research on the application of shiatsu to various aspects of maternity care. It is also worthwhile referring to the NHS CRD review (2001), which is an overview of all acupuncture studies.

Analgesia in labour

The area which has been most researched is analgesia. Indeed, it was this field which first brought acupuncture to public attention. A large study in China analysed two groups of women having Caesareans: one group containing 24 271 cases from 1975 to 1980 in 18 provinces and the other containing 16 649 cases from 1981 to 1987 in five provinces. The success rates were 92.1% and 98.9%, and the combined rates of excellent and good degrees were 74.5% and 87.1%, respectively. It concluded that acupuncture anaesthesia could be a good anaesthetic method for Caesarean section (Wang & Jin 1989).

Shiatsu has long been used for analgesia in Japan. A small study was done in 1962 by Dr T. Utsugi, head of the obstetrics and gynecology department of the Japan Red Cross Hospital at Kasaoka, Okayama Prefecture; he achieved a high average of 93.3% of painless labour by giving a special treatment of shiatsu and massage where pressure was applied to the coccyx, waist and inguinal regions (Utsugi, unpublished work, 2001). A study is currently underway in the Western Galilee Hospital on the benefits of shiatsu for labour (Utsugi & Noe, unpublished work, 2002).

Many studies have been done on acupuncture, some of which include electro-acupuncture, acupressure and needles. Some studies have been done where midwives who have undergone short training courses have been able to achieve benefits. One such study involving a small trial of 90 women showed a reduction in the need for epidurals and better relaxation with no negative effects (Ramnero et al 2001). Another study in Cyprus using ear and hand points showed high apgar (9.6 at 1 min) with slight to good results in 87.5% cases (Martoudis & Christofides 1990). An English study of 85 women receiving acupuncture reported their feelings of calmness and well-being and of being in control of their own labour and delivery; this did not necessarily correlate with a marked decrease of pain relief. However, there was evidence that acupuncture resulted in a shorter first stage of labour (Skelton & Flowerdew 1988). Other studies have supported the analgesic effects of acupuncture without adverse effects (Arkatov et al 1992, Ceccherelli et al 1996, Kvorning Ternov et al 1998, Oberg et al 1991, White 1999). One Russian study (Oberg et al 1991) found the abolishment of preliminary pain sensations, normalization of central nervous system function, autonomic reactions, uterine contractility, a reduction in pharmacological agent use and treatment duration, and better delivery.

A couple of studies did not find such a positive effect, although one Nigerian study still felt that although the results were inconsistent and unpredictable, the simplicity, cheapness and absence of physiological complications make it a worth-while medical armament for pain relief in the Nigerian environment, with limited resources and specialized manpower (sic) (Umeh 1986). The other study of 32 primiparous women who had received repeated treatment with acupuncture during the month prior to term found that acupuncture did not reduce the need for analgesics in labour (Lyrenas et al 1990).

Some studies have tried to investigate how the analgesic affect is achieved. One study suggested that acupuncture may reduce the content of substance P in the serum of the gravida (Ma et al 1992).

A massage study of 28 women found that massage therapy during the first 15 min of each hour of childbirth decreased anxiety and pain, as well as the need for medication and the length of labour (Field et al 1997).

Induction and augmentation of labour

There have been many studies on this although the Cochrane Review found no randomized controlled trials which met all their inclusion criteria and concluded that there is a need for a well designed randomized controlled trial to evaluate the role of acupuncture to induce labour (Smith & Crowther 2002).

A small study was done in Australia using the points SP-6 and LV-3 which showed an increased frequency of higher intensity contractions, although no women went into labour (Dunn et al 1989). Other studies have indicated the uses of acupuncture in inducing labour and increasing the strength of contractions (Kubista et al 1975, Malkov Ialu Biserova 1989, Rabl et al 2001, Tsuei et al 1974).

A dramatic study in Yunnan, China, using volunteers who had applied for abortion or induction of labour found that needling Hegu (LI-4) and Sanyinjiao (SP-6) could initiate uterine contractions at any stage of pregnancy, including first term (Li 1981). One very small study (five women) indicated that labour was rapidly induced, although pain wasn't affected, and the length of labour was shorter (Ricci 1997). Another study found that first stage was shorter (Lin 1998). Another used ear acupuncture to dilate the cervix for abortion in cases where, because of the tightness of the cervical os, artificial abortion and diagnostic curettage had proved impossible (Zhang & Lu 1984).

A study on rats showed the opposite effect i.e. stopping pre-term labour. Acupuncture on LI-4 was found to suppress uterine contractions induced by oxytocin in the pregnant rat. If acupuncture is similarly effective in counteracting the effects of oxytocin in women, then this may be an alternative medical treatment for women in pre-term labour (Pak et al 2000). This is interesting as it shows that points work to support the body to do what it needs to do – i.e. if it needs to go into labour, then using certain points will enable the body to move into labour, if the body needs to stop going into labour then the use of the same points will stop labour. It is an indication of the safety.

Other effects on labour – length, normality of contractions, postpartum haemorrhage

One study showed that acupuncture shortens the length of the first stage, 196 min compared with 321 min in the group without acupuncture (Zeisler et al 1998).

Another study used acupuncture of LI-4 to reduce the second stage of labour and postpartum haemorrhage (Shang et al 1995). Although one study of 56 women concluded that it may lengthen pregnancy and labour, looking at the figures it was only 0.3 h longer for the second stage and the first stage was shorter (Lyrenas et al 1987). Another study found that acupuncture encouraged the process of normal labour in a group of 80 women at risk of developing labour activity abnormalities, as well as reducing blood loss, and was conducive to improvement of autonomic nervous system activity with the predominance of the cholinergic component (Aleksandrina et al 1992). A retrospective study showed acupuncture to be an effective, simple and safe method for retained placenta (Chauhan et al 1998).

Pregnancy benefits

Many benefits have been demonstrated in pregnancy.

Fetal presentation

Several studies have been done on correcting fetal presentation, all of which indicate promising results (Wang et al 1998). One demonstrated a success rate of 83.3% – remarkably higher than treatment by knee–chest positioning (Qin & Tang 1989). In another, 24 subjects in the control group and one subject in the intervention group underwent external cephalic version, but at term 98 (75.4%) of the 130 fetuses in the intervention group were cephalic at birth vs 81 (62.3%) of the 130 fetuses in the control group (Cardini & Weixin 1998).

Treatment of nausea and morning sickness

Recently, three good studies have been carried out in this area (Carlsson et al 2000, Smith et al 2002, Steele et al 2001). One studied 593 women who were less than 14 weeks pregnant in a single blind randomized controlled trial (RCT) in Australia and concluded that acupuncture is an effective treatment for women who experience nausea and dry retching in early pregnancy (Smith et al 2002). Another was also a carefully designed RCT and noted a significant benefit in manual acupuncture in reducing hyperemesis gravidarum. The treatment placebo group were not entirely placebo but near placebo. No side effects were observed during or after the study (Carlsson et al 2000).

Prior to this, many studies have been done on the effects of acupressure and acupuncture which have shown positive results (Bayreuther et al 1994, Belluomini et al 1994, De Aloysio & Penacchioni 1992, Dundee et al 1988, Norheim et al 2001, Stainton & Neff 1994). The Cochrane Review (Jewell & Young 2002) felt they were equivocal and that more studies were needed, although there was no evidence of teratogenicity. Some studies that found positive effects were poorly designed or subjective (Cong-lian 1999, Dundee 1988, Hyde 1989, Rongjun 1987). Two studies showed no benefit (Knight et al 2001, O'Brien et al 1996). Vickers also provides a review of research in this area (Vickers 1996).

There have been some studies that have looked at using acupressure for reducing nausea during and after Caesarean section which indicate a possible benefit (Duggal et al 1998, Harmon et al 2000, Ho et al 1996, Stein et al 1997).

Other pregnancy benefits including relief of back pain

There is some evidence for other benefits of massage and shiatsu in pregnancy. A study of 26 women having massage for 20 min twice a week showed decreased anxiety and a decreased level of stress hormones (norepinephrine) during pregnancy, and reduced anxiety, improved mood, better sleep, less back pain and fewer obstetric and postnatal complications including lower prematurity rates (Field et al 1999). Another showed similar benefits for depressed mothers (Field et al, in preparation).

A case study has been presented showing the benefit of acupuncture for chronic pelvic pain at 27 weeks' gestation: normal delivery followed (Napolitano 2000). There has been research on the benefits of massage and shiatsu in the reduction of back pain in non-pregnant clients (Brady et al 2001, Hernandez-Reif et al 2001), which indicates its uses in pregnant clients. A study on acupuncture for back pain has also been concluded (Wedenbegh et al 2000).

Babies

According to Cochrane, the evidence that massage for preterm infants has a beneficial effect on developmental outcomes is weak (Vickers et al 2002) but some studies have indicated there may be benefits which would be worthy of further research (Harrison et al 2000) such as weight gain (Dieter et al, submitted), more optimal cognitive and motor development (Field et al 1987) and better sleep patterns (Scafadi et al 1986). A study indicated that massage can alleviate stress in newborns in special care (Field 1990), while another demonstrated that touch is not harmful for the preterm as some previously thought (Adamson-Macedo et al 1997).

With newborns, one study showed that massage with oil has more positive effects (Field et al 1996b). Others show that bonding and involvement of fathers can be improved (Cullen et al 2000, Scholtz & Samuels 1992). A study on the infants of depressed mothers showed that after the massage they slept more, but overall spent more time in active alert and active awake states, cried less, and had lower salivary cortisol levels, suggesting lower stress; they also showed a greater improvement on emotionality, sociability and soothability temperament dimensions and had greater decreases in urinary stress catecholamines/hormones (norepinephrine, epinephrine, cortisol) (Field et al 1996a).

One study reviewed the data on the effects of massage therapy on infants and children with various medical conditions, including infants who were: premature, cocaine and HIV exposed, parented by depressed mothers, and full-term infants without medical problems. The childhood conditions included: abuse (sexual and physical), asthma, autism, burns, cancer, developmental delays, dermatitis (psoriasis), diabetes, eating disorders (bulimia), juvenile rheumatoid arthritis, post-traumatic stress disorder and psychiatric problems. Generally, the massage therapy resulted in lower anxiety and stress hormones and an improved clinical course. Having grandparent volunteers and parents give the therapy enhances their own wellness and provides a cost effective treatment for the children (Field 1995).

Another study reviewed massage on neonates born to HIV-positive mothers and found a superior performance on almost every Brazelton newborn cluster score; the neonates had a greater daily weight gain at the end of the treatment period unlike the control group who showed declining performance (Scafidi & Field 1996).

Safety issues

From the numerous studies carried out over many years, none have given rise to any concern over safety issues. This is confirmed by the NHS CRD review (2001). Indeed, even in Western culture, there are references on the safety and effectiveness of massage which date back to Plato. As shiatsu is about rebalancing the body's own energy and not putting anything into it, there are not the same kind of safety issues as with drugs and technology. For someone to be 'harmed' by shiatsu, they have to be worked in a way that doesn't feel comfortable. The risks involved are to do with overly strong manipulation of the body or a lack of understanding of basic anatomy and physiology. In terms of looking at potential side effects, the only cases that have come to light serve to illustrate this point.

A letter was signed by three doctors from US medical schools and concerned the case of a 61-year-old physician who underwent a professional shiatsu massage. The day after shiatsu, the recipient noticed 'painless weakness of the left thumb, without sensory symptoms'. Medical examination suggested 'isolated dysfunction of the recurrent thenar motor branch of the median nerve, apparently the result of focal trauma from the massage'. The symptoms improved after 3 weeks and normalized over the next few months. There was no direct evidence that the shiatsu caused the injury (Herskovitz et al 1992).

The other case was about a 31-year-old woman in California who, in an attempt to avoid asthma attacks she had experienced in previous pregnancies, tried acupuncture. She soon developed bilateral pneumothoraces, and of the four previously reported cases following acupuncture one proved fatal. The point needled was probably Lung 1 and it is clearly stated in acupuncture texts (Deadman & Al-Khafaji 1998) that a caution for this point is 'deep perpendicular or oblique insertion carries a substantial risk of causing a pneumothorax' (Anon 1991).

I do not feel that it is possible to make a list of absolute contraindications because the situations in which shiatsu is sometimes listed as contraindicated relate either to areas where shiatsu needs to be carried out alongside a Western approach (such as infection, inflammation, cancer, pre-eclampsia, thrombosis) or where knowledge of the relevant physiology will guide the correct use of shiatsu such as in infections (not to work in a stimulating way), thrombosis and veins (not to work directly over the area).

The body does give immediate feedback. The shiatsu outlined in this book does not involve the use of strong manipulative techniques, mainly because they are not suitable for the pregnant body which is softened by increased levels of relaxin and progesterone. These types of techniques are also not shown because they require advanced body skill knowledge and need to be learnt directly from an experienced teacher.

Summary

There is enough research on shiatsu to support its use in a variety of situations, providing that the midwife has been properly trained and pays attention to the relevant professional and employment issues.

Points for reflection

Think about how you want to use or are using shiatsu in your practice and consider how you are going to address all the relevant issues.

REFERENCES

Adamson-Macedo E N, de Roiste A, Wilson A et al 1997 Systematic gentle/light stroking and maternal random touching of ventilated preterm: a preliminary study. International Journal of Prenatal and Perinatal Psychology and Medicine 9(1):17–31

Aleksandrina E V, Zharkin A F, Gavrilova A S 1992 [The acupuncture prevention of anomalies in labor strength in pregnant women of a risk group.] Akusherstvo i ginekologiia (Mosk) (8–12):22–24

Allaire A D, Moos M K, Wells S R 2000 Complementary and alternative medicine in pregnancy: a survey of North Carolina certified nurse-midwives. Obstetrics and Gynecology (Jan) 95(1):19–23

American College of Nurse Midwives 1993 Core competences for basic midwifery practice. Guidelines for Incorporation of New Procedures into Midwifery Practice. American College of Nurse Midwives, USA

Anon 1991 Pop goes the needle. Lancet 337(8737):355–356

Arkatov V A, Zverev V V, Volkovinskii K E 1992 [The effect of tramal and acupuncture analgesia on labor pain and the psychoemotional status of the parturient.] Anesteziologiia i reanimatologiia Mar–Apr (2):31–33

Ballegaard S, Norrelund S, Smith D F 1996 Cost-benefit of combined use of acupuncture, shiatsu and lifestyle adjustment for treatment of patients with severe angina pectoris. Acupuncture and Electro-therapeutics Research 21(3–4):187–197

Bayreuther J, Lewith G T, Pickering R 1994 A double-blind cross-over study to evaluate the effectiveness of acupressure at pericardium 6 (p6) in the treatment of early morning sickness (EMS). Complementary Therapies in Medicine 2:70–76

Belluomini J, Litt R C, Lee K A et al 1994 Acupressure for nausea and vomiting of pregnancy: a randomized, blinded study. Obstetrics and Gynecology 84(2):245–248

Bensoussan A 1991 The vital meridian. Churchill Livingstone, Edinburgh

Brady L H, Henry K, Luth J F et al 2001 The effects of shiatsu on lower back pain. Journal of Holistic Nursing 19(1):57–70

British Medical Association 1993 Complementary medicine, new approaches to good practice. Oxford University Press, Oxford

Burns E, Blamey C, Llody A J 2000 Aromatherapy in childbirth: an effective approach to care. British Journal of Midwifery 8(10):639–643

Cardini F, Weixin H 1998 Moxibustion for correction of breech presentation: a randomized controlled trial. Journal of the American Medical Association Nov 11 280(18):1580–1584

Carlsson C P O, Axemo P, Bodin A 2000 Manual acupuncture reduces hyperemesis gravidarum: a placebo-controlled, randomised, single blind, crossover study. Journal of Pain and Symptom Management 20(4):273–279

Ceccherelli F, Gagliardi G, Giugni G M et al 1996 Techniche di iperstimolazione nel trattamento del dolore travaglio di parto. Rassegna della letteratura. Giornale Italiano di Riflessoterapia ed Agopunctura 8(2–3):165–173

Chauhan P A, Gasser F J, Chauhan A M 1998 Clinical investigation on the use of acupuncture for treatment of placental retention. American Journal of Acupuncture 26(1):19–25

Cheesman S, Christian R, Cresswell J 2001 Exploring the value of shiatsu in palliative care day services. International Journal of Palliative Nursing 7(5):234–239

Cong-lian Z 1999 Acupuncture for vomitus gravidarum. International Journal of Clinical Acupuncture 10(3):335–336

Cullen C, Field T, Escalona A et al 2000 Father–infants interactions are enhanced by massage therapy. Early Child Development and Care 164:41–47

Deadman P, Al-Khafaji M 1998 Manual of acupuncture. Journal of Chinese Medicine Publications, Hove

De Aloysio D, Penacchioni P 1992 Morning sickness control in early pregnancy by Neiguan point acupressure. Obstetrics and Gynecology 80(5):852–854

Department of Health 2000 Complementary medicine: information for primary care clinicians. Department of Health, Foundation for integrated medicine and NHS Alliance, London

Duggal K N, Douglas M J, Peter E A et al 1998 Acupressure for intrathecal narcotic-induced nausea and vomiting after caesarean section. International Journal of Obstetric Anesthesia 7(4):231–236

Dundee J 1988 Acupuncture/acupressure as an antiemetic: studies of its use in postoperative vomiting, cancer chemotherapy and sickness of early pregnancy. Complementary Medical Research 3(1):2–14

Dundee J W, Sourial F B R, Ghaly R G 1988 P6 acupuncture reduces morning sickness. Journal of the Royal Society of Medicine 81(8):456–457

Dunn P A, App M, Rogers D et al 1989 Transcutaneous electrical nerve stimulation at acupuncture points in the induction of uterine contractions. Obstetrics and Gynecology 73(2):286–290

Field T 1990 Alleviating stress in newborn infants in the intensive care unit. Perinatology 17:1–9

Field T 1995 Massage therapy for infants and children. Journal of Developmental & Behavioral Pediatrics 16:105–111

Field T, Scafidi F A, Schanberg S et al 1987 Massage of preterm newborns to improve growth and development. Pediatric Nursing 13:385–387

Field T, Grizzle N, Scafidi F et al 1996a Massage therapy for infants of depressed mothers. Infant Behavior and Development 19:109–114

Field T, Schanberg S, Davalos M et al 1996b Massage with oil has more positive effects on newborn infants. Pre and Perinatal Psychology Journal 11:73–78

Field T, Hernandez-Reif M, Taylor S et al 1997 Labor pain is reduced by massage therapy. Journal of Psychosomatic Obstetrics and Gynaecology 18(4):286–291

Field T, Hernandez-Reif M, Hart S et al 1999 Pregnant women benefit from massage therapy. Journal of Psychosomatic Obstetrics and Gynecology 20(1):31–38

Harmon D, Ryan M, Kelly A et al 2000 Acupressure and prevention of nausea and vomiting during and after spinal anaesthesia for caesarean section. British Journal of Anaesthesia 84(4):463–467

Harrison L L, Williams A K, Berbaum M L et al 2000 Effects of developmental, health status, behavioral, and environmental variables on preterm infants' responses to a gentle human touch intervention. International Journal of Prenatal and Perinatal Psychology and Medicine 12(1):109–122

Hernandez-Reif M, Field T, Krasnegor J et al 2001 Low back pain is reduced and range of motion increased after massage therapy. International Journal of Neuroscience 106:131–145

Herskovitz S, Strauch B, Gordon M J V 1992 Shiatsu massage-induced injury of the median recurrent motor branch (letter). Muscle & Nerve 15(10):1215

Ho C, Hseu S, Tsai S et al 1996 Effects of P6 acupressure on prevention of nausea and vomiting after epidural morphine for post-caesarean section pain relief. Acta Anaesthesia Scandinavia 40:371–375

Hodnett E D 2002 Support from caregivers during childbirth. Cochrane Review in Cochrane Library, Issue 3, Update Software Ltd, Oxford

Hyde E 1989 Acupressure therapy for morning sickness. A controlled clinical trial. Journal of Nurse Midwifery 34(4):171–178

Jewell D, Young G 2002 Interventions for nausea and vomiting in early pregnancy. Cochrane Review in Cochrane Library, Issue 2, Update Software Ltd, Oxford

Knight B, Mudge C, Openshaw S et al 2001 Effect of acupuncture on nausea of pregnancy: a randomized, controlled trial. Obstetrics and Gynecology 97(2):184–188

Kubista E, Kucera H, Muller E 1975 Initiating contractions of the gravid uterus through electroacupuncture. American Journal of Chinese Medicine 3(4):343–346

Kvorning Ternov N, Buchhave P, Svensson G et al 1998 Acupuncture during childbirth reduces use of conventional analgesia without major adverse effects: a retrospective study. American Journal of Acupuncture 26(4):233–239

Li H F 1981 The effect of puncturing the Hegu and Sanyinjiao points in pregnancy. Yunnan Journal of Traditional Chinese Medicine 6:33

Lin P C 1998 Acupuncture to accelerate labor. International Journal of Clinical Acupuncture 9(4):459–462

Lloyd P, Lupton D, Wiesner D et al 1993 Choosing alternative therapy: an exploratory study of sociodemographic characteristics and motive of patients resident in Sydney. Australian Journal of Public Health 17(2):135–144

Lynch B 2002 Keynote speech. Care for the caregiver. International Confederation of Midwives Conference, Vienna

Lyrenas S, Lutsch H, Hetta J et al 1987 Acupuncture before delivery: effect on labor. Gynecol Obstet Invest 24(4):217–224

Lyrenas S, Lutsch H, Hetta J et al 1990 Acupuncture before delivery: effect on pain perception and the need for analgesics. Gynecologic and Obstetric Investigation 29(2):118–124

Ma H, Jiang E, Zhao X 1992 The effect of acupuncture on the content of substance P in serum of gravida during delivery. Chen Tzu Yen Chiu 17(1):65–66

McCabe P 2001 Complementary therapies in nursing and midwifery. Ausmed Publications, Melbourne, Australia

Malkov IaIu Biserova N N 1989 [Uterine contractile activity in parturients of a group at risk for prolonged pregnancy prepared for labor by acupuncture reflexotherapy.] Akusherstvo i ginekologiia (Mosk) Nov (11):30–34

Martoudis S G, Christofides K 1990 Electroacupuncture for pain relief in labour. Acupuncture in Medicine 8(2):51–53

Napolitano P G 2000 Use of acupuncture for managing chronic pelvic pain in pregnancy: a case report. Journal of Reproductive Medicine for the Obstetrician and Gynecologist 45(11):944–946

NHS Centre for reviews (CRD) 2001 Effective health care – acupuncture. 7(2)

Norheim A J, Pedersen E J, Fonnebo V et al 2001 Acupressure treatment of morning sickness in pregnancy. Scandinavian Journal of Primary Health Care 19:43–47

Nurses Board of Victoria, Australia 1999 Guidelines for use of complementary therapies in nursing practice. Nurses Board of Victoria, Melbourne, Australia

Nursing and Midwifery Council 2002 Code of professional conduct. Nursing and Midwifery Council, London

Oberg O K, Shatkina G V, Slavutskaia M V et al 1991 [Reflex analgesia in the combined treatment of pregnant women with a pathological preliminary period.] Akusherstvo i ginekologiia (Mosk) Feb (2):37–39

O'Brien B, Relyea J, Taerum T 1996 Efficacy of P6 acupressure in the treatment of nausea and vomiting during pregnancy. American Journal of Obstetrics and Gynecology 174(2):708–715

Pak S C, Na C S, Kim J S et al 2000 The effect of acupuncture on uterine contraction induced by oxytocin. American Journal of Chinese Medicine 28(1):35–40

Qin G F, Tang H J 1989 413 cases of abnormal fetal position corrected by auricular plaster therapy.

Journal of Traditional Chinese Medicine Dec 9(4): 235–237

Ramnero A, Hanson U, Kihlgren M 2001 Acupuncture treatment during childbirth – a randomised trial. Presented at the International Confederation of Midwives conference, Vienna, March 2002

Ricci L 1997 Agopunctura per l'induzione e l'analgesia nel travaglio di parto (5 casi). Giornale Italiano di Riflessoterapia ed Agopunctura 9(2):105–107

Rongjun Z 1987 39 Cases of morning sickness treated with acupuncture. Journal of Traditional Chinese Medicine 7(1):25–26

Royal College of Medicine 1999 Position Paper No. 10a: Complementary therapies. RCM Midwives Journal 2(12):382–384

Scafidi F, Field T 1996 Massage therapy improves behavior in neonates born to HIV-positive mothers. Journal of Pediatric Psychology 21:889–897

Scafidi F, Field T, Schanberg S et al 1986 Effects of tactile/kinesthetic stimulation on the clinical course and sleep/wake behavior of preterm neonates. Infant Behavior and Development 9:91–105

Scholtz K, Samuels C A 1992 Neonatal bathing and massage intervention with fathers, behavioural effects 12 weeks after birth of the first baby: The Sunraysia Australia Intervention Project. International Journal of Behavioral Development 15:67–81

Shang L F, Liu J Y, Li A X 1995 [Puncture of the Hegu acupoint to accelerate the second stage of labor and to reduce postpartum hemorrhage.] Chung Hua Hu Li Tsa Chih Sep 5 30(9):537–538

Skelton I F, Flowerdew M W 1988 Acupuncture and labour – a summary of results. Midwives Chronicle and Nursing Notes (May) 101(1204):134–138

Smith C A, Crowther C A 2002 Acupuncture for induction of labour. Cochrane Review in Cochrane Library, Issue 2, Update Software Ltd, Oxford

Smith C, Crowther C, Beilby J 2002 Acupuncture to treat nausea and vomiting in early pregnancy: a randomized controlled trial. Birth 29(1):1–9

Stainton M C, Neff E J A 1994 The efficacy of SeaBands for the control of nausea and vomiting in pregnancy. Health Care for Women International 15(6):563–575

Steele N M, French J, Gatherer-Boyles J et al 2001 Effect of acupressure by sea-bands on nausea and vomiting of pregnancy. Journal of Obstetric, Gynecologic, and Neonatal Nursing 30(1):61–70

Stein D J, Birnbach D J, Danzer B I et al 1997 Acupressure versus intravenous metoclopramide to prevent nausea and vomiting during spinal anesthesia for cesarean section. Anesthesia and Analgesia 84(2):342–345

Tiran D, Mack S 1995 Complementary therapies for pregnancy and childbirth. Bailliere Tindall, London

Tsuei J J, Lai F, Lai Y-L 1974 Induction of labour by acupuncture and electrical stimulation. Obstetrics and Gynaecology 43(3):337

Umeh B U 1986 Sacral acupuncture for pain relief in labour: initial clinical experience in Nigerian women. Acupuncture and Electro-therapeutics Research 11(2):147–151

United Kingdom Central Council 1998 Midwives' Rules and Code of Practice, UKCC, London

Vickers A J 1996 Can acupuncture have specific effects on health – a systematic review of acupuncture anti-emesis RCTs. Journal of the Royal Society of Medicine 89:303–311

Vickers A, Ohlsson A, Lacy J B et al 2002 Massage for promoting growth and development of preterm and/or low birth-weight infants. Cochrane Review in Cochrane Library, Issue 2, Update Software Ltd, Oxford

Wang D W, Jin Y H 1989 Present status of cesarean section under acupuncture anesthesia in China.

Fukushima Journal of Medical Science 35(2):45–52

Wang Z, Wang X X, Wang S Y 1998 Correction of pelvic presentation by magnetic bead attached to ear points: a clinical report of 45 cases. International Journal of Clinical Acupuncture 9(2):221–223

Wedenbegh K, Moen B, Noling A 2000 A prospective randomised study comparing acupuncture with physiotherapy for low back and pelvic pain in pregnancy. Acta Obstet Gyncol Scand 79:331–335

White A R 1999 Acupuncture may help those who choose it for childbirth. Focus on Alternative and Complementary Therapies Jun 4(2):65

Zeisler H, Tempfer C, Mayerhofer K et al 1998 Influence of acupuncture on duration of labor. Gynecologic and Obstetric Investigation 46(1):22–25

Zhang H Y, Yu L H 1984 Observations on the effect of auriculo-acupuncture for dilatation of cervical os in 56 cases. Second National Symposium of Acupuncture, Moxibustion and Acupuncture Anaesthesia. Paper No 87 Beijing.

Yin and Yang – applying Eastern theory to midwifery

'Shiatsu no kokoro wa haha gokoro' – 'The heart of shiatsu is mother's love' (Tokujiro Namikoshi)

The main purpose of this section is to provide a cohesive theoretical description, from a shiatsu point of view, of what is happening to the mother and baby in the antenatal, intrapartum and postnatal periods. It offers a different view from the conventional Western approach. It explains how shiatsu works so that midwives can understand the main ways in which to work and why. You may not understand all the concepts on the first reading, but it should provide a useful reference tool so that, as you use shiatsu, you will gradually understand more of these concepts. When reading the practical section (Section 3) you can look back to here to understand more about why you need to work with certain meridians. The other purpose of this section is to describe how shiatsu has been used in Japan both historically and in the present time. It will also describe the uses of shiatsu in other countries outside Japan, primarily focusing on its use in the UK, but including examples worldwide. Chapter 3 explores the nature of Chinese medical theory, its underpinning beliefs and key concepts. Chapter 4 looks more specifically at how these concepts are applied to form an understanding of the antenatal, intrapartum and postnatal periods.

3

Key concepts

Introduction

Shiatsu theory developed from traditional Chinese medical theory which arrived in Japan around the 6th century AD. It is likely, even before this, in common with most traditional cultures, that some form of healing through touch existed. Many people suggest that a form of shiatsu predates acupuncture even in China itself.

Shiatsu developed in Japan through being practised, blending the Chinese theoretical concepts with existing knowledge and skills. In Japan there was a particular emphasis on the importance of ampuku – massage of the hara or abdomen.

Originally, shiatsu was a form of massage known as amna which was often practised by the blind. The term shiatsu was first used by Tamia Tempaku, an amna practitioner, in 1915 in his book 'Shiatsu Ryoho' (Tempaku 1915). By the 1920s, it had degenerated into being mainly a massage for pleasure and relaxation, used in the court and the bath houses by the 'shampooers', although it was still widely used by the traditional midwives (known as 'sambas'). In 1925, the Shiatsu Therapists Association was formed to promote amna as a remedial therapy, calling it 'shiatsu'. Tokujiro Namikoshi, its founder and a student of Tempaku, wanted to place shiatsu in a Western framework. He tended to favour a Western scientific approach over classical theory, although he expressed the importance of shiatsu as a way of emotionally connecting through touch, coining the phrase, still known today in Japan, 'Shiatsu no kokoro wa haha gokoro' ('the heart of shiatsu is mother's love').

After the Second World War and the American occupation of Japan, shiatsu was temporarily banned by General McArthur. Although shiatsu was rapidly reinstated, with the intercession of

---

Case study 3.1   Ikuyo Hosaka – a samba who practised shiatsu in her work and whose knowledge is passed on in this book

Ikuyo was born in 1917 and originally trained as a nurse from 1933 to 1936. In 1940, with two young daughters, one a baby, she decided to train as a midwife so she would have a more secure job if her husband died in the war. She lived in the countryside of Yamanashi and had to do a 6-month samba training and sit for the state examination along with women who were mostly traditional midwives and not nurses like her. In 1941 she went to the local Red Cross Hospital, where she had previously worked as nurse, for 10 days to get her clinical practice. In those 10 days she attended 10 births and was 'ready' for practice. For her first birth a few days later, she was called to the mountains to attend a woman who at 30, extremely old for those days, was giving birth to her first baby. She had been in labour for three nights and three days and had ruptured membranes for one day. When Ikuyo arrived, the head was coming but the baby was flat. Ikuyo had to resuscitate the baby mouth to mouth for 30 min but eventually the baby cried and recovered. Her first wage was a bowl of white rice – a luxury. Eventually she set up a birth house in her home, starting with three and growing to nine beds. In her career she attended over 5000 births.

Ikuyo used shiatsu a great deal in her work – during most births she would use some shiatsu. She never did any formal training but picked it up from the knowledge around her – family, friends and probably through her contacts with the traditional non-nurse trained midwives. An educated woman, she also would study texts on points and add new knowledge to her work. Her daughter and granddaughter both trained as midwives and it is through her granddaughter, Naoko Natsume, who now works as an independent midwife in London, that I have learnt about her work. Unfortunately, Ikuyo died in 1987 before Naoko had a chance to study directly from her, but Naoko has pieced together Ikuyo's knowledge through her self-published book 'My half-life record' (published in 1978) and fragments of her diaries (Naoko Natsume, personal communication). Section 3 of this book will refer to points and techniques that Ikuyo used.

---

the American champion of blind causes, Helen Keller, the traditional role of the sambas was diminished by the medicalization of birth. Almost overnight, the situation whereby most women gave birth at home or in midwives' houses changed, so that more births took place in the new American-style hospitals. By 1960 it was official – the safest place to give birth was hospital.

This was accompanied by a change in midwifery training. Until 1947 sambas had their own specific midwifery course. After 1947 they came under the umbrella of nursing and health visiting and had first to train as a nurse. The newly trained midwives were renamed 'josanpu'. The traditional shiatsu skills of the sambas were rapidly lost and today only a handful of elderly sambas or independent midwives still use their knowledge (Takahashi 1996).

Shizuto Masunaga became one of the most important shiatsu practitioners and teachers in the 1960s and 1970s until his death in 1981. His mother had studied shiatsu and Masunaga studied at the Namikoshi school, and taught there for 10 years. He then set up his own school, the Iokai Centre in Tokyo. His contribution was to blend psychology and Western physiology with orthodox shiatsu practice in an approach known as Zen shiatsu (Masunaga 1977, 1987).

In Japan today both Masunaga's and Namikoshi's schools, along with many other shiatsu schools still exist. There were 96 788 registered shiatsu and amna practitioners in Japan in 2000 compared with 24 511 midwives (Health Statistics Office 2000). This impressive figure doesn't mean that shiatsu is widely used in Japan. This number represents all the people who have studied the state examination for the professional qualification in shiatsu. Most of these then go on to practise Western massage such as sports

---

Table 3.1   National statistics for place of birth, Japan (Maternal and Child Health Statistics of Japan 2001)

	1950	1960	1970	2000
Hospital birth	2.9% (including hospital, clinic, maternity home = 4.6%)	24.1% (including hospital, clinic, maternity home = 50.1%)	43.3% (including hospital, clinic, maternity home = 96.1%)	53.7% (including hospital, clinic, maternity home = 99.8%)
Maternity home	0.5%	8.5%	10.6%	1.0%
Home birth	95.4%	49.9%	3.9%	0.2%

massage, beauty therapy or aromatherapy. Shiatsu in its remedial form is not widely used in Japan today. Most people will first consult a doctor trained in Western medicine which is covered by health insurance whereas shiatsu usually is not. Antenatally, most women will go to their doctor who may well be suspicious of shiatsu. Not many women will have shiatsu during their pregnancy. People might know of a specific shiatsu point for headaches or backache and may even work some points on themselves, but do not use it much beyond that.

Both Masunaga's and Namikoshi's style influenced the development of shiatsu outside Japan which began to occur from the 1970s onwards. It first spread to America as some of its teachers, notably Waturu Ohashi (Ohashi 1977) and Pauline Sasaki, moved from Japan to live and teach there. Shortly afterwards, it spread to the UK and Europe. The Shiatsu Society was established in the UK in 1981 to support the development of shiatsu as a profession in the UK. The Shiatsu Society holds a register of practitioners and supports training and professional regulation. Gradually, a system of schools with a 3-year training programme has developed in the UK. In Canada, USA, Australia, New Zealand and throughout Europe there are similar associations supporting the development of shiatsu as a profession (see Appendix 2).

Unfortunately, since 1944, there has not been much emphasis on the role of shiatsu in maternity care, as the knowledge of the sambas has become hidden. This book will draw together their empirical knowledge with my own work in the field since 1989, to provide a cohesive approach to the antenatal, intrapartum and postnatal periods. The theory in this chapter is drawn from my own studies, initially in the Masunaga system but later drawing more directly upon traditional Chinese knowledge. For this, I am particularly indebted to the work of Giovanni Maciocia (Maciocia 1989, 1998).

The theory is in a sense a metaphor to describe something that in essence is very simple – a knowledge of the body as understood primarily through the hands. It is tempting to think of the Eastern system as something alien and different, but it is simply another way of looking at the human body. The main difference between the traditional Eastern and Western body map is that the Eastern view always looks at the whole, whereas the West splits it into parts. The two systems can ultimately link together to give a complete picture of the body.

The Eastern 'meridian map' of energy – key concepts in shiatsu

The whole in a state of constant change

> 'One Infinity differentiates into Yin and Yang, which begin a spirallic inward process of physical and material manifestation through the continuously transforming worlds of vibration or energy, pre-atomic particles, elements, vegetable life and animal life of which man (sic) is the last result. Upon becoming human, we then start to return to One Infinity through an expanding spiral of decomposition and spiritualisation, melting personal and individual identities' (Kushi 1977).

Shiatsu has its theoretical origins in the East, thousands of years ago, when the world view was of everything being part of a whole, known as the Tao. The ancient Chinese saw humans as expressions of this whole – microcosms of the universe. The universe included the solar system as well as the earth but this book will only consider in detail their theories about the earth. While theories about the human body were being developed, people lived more in contact with the rhythms of nature, than we do today. This can help explain an early difference between what later developed into Eastern and Western philosophies. In ancient China and Japan, nature was seen as a supportive and positive system – unlike in the ancient Middle East, the homeland of modern Western philosophies, where nature was seen as harsh and something to be controlled. The human body fitted into this system not as a static entity, but, like the world in which we live, always in a constant state of change. The body was considered as being rather like a garden, subject to different rhythms according both to the time of the day and the seasons.

The traditions of healing which developed were to do with nurturing and supporting these bodily rhythms. The Chinese considered the body as an expression of the Tao, the whole. The physical structure and the emotional and spiritual aspects of the body are all interconnected. Each can only be seen as part of the whole and considered in relationship to the whole. If a mother is sick in pregnancy, it is seen as being caused by different aspects of her body's energy being out of balance and this needs to be addressed in order for the sickness to subside. In pregnancy, the baby is seen as being part of the mother's energy system and after birth the mother's energy will continue to affect the baby profoundly, especially while she is still breastfeeding.

As soon as a change is made in one part of the body this has a direct effect on all other parts of the body. The view of health is where the body as a whole is in harmony. If areas of the body are not in harmony then balance needs to be restored. There are various ways of doing this, and shiatsu is just one of them. This balance is not static but expresses itself as a movement of energy between the two opposing poles of Yin and Yang.

Yin and Yang

Daily movement of energy

The whole expresses itself in a multitude of ways. Yin and Yang represent the most basic movement of energy in the earth, which is the movement from night to day. The Chinese used their writing or characters to express many levels of meaning and these often relate to nature. Yin is represented by the Chinese character for the shady side of the mountain and Yang is the sunny side of the mountain (Fig. 3.1). Yang is about energy moving outwards and Yin is about energy moving inwards; they are not, as people sometimes mistakenly say, active and passive energies. From this, we get the qualities associated with Yin of being dark, cold, hidden, slower, quieter, and of Yang being bright, hot, revealed, faster, louder.

This daily movement of energy expresses clearly the qualities of Yin and Yang, and is also expressed in the Taoist symbol (Fig. 3.2).

Certain principles can be drawn from the characters of Yin and Yang:

1. Yin and Yang exist only in relation to each other. Day cannot exist without night.

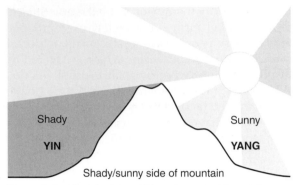

Figure 3.1   Yin (shady) and Yang (sunny) sides of the mountain – the literal representation of the Chinese character.

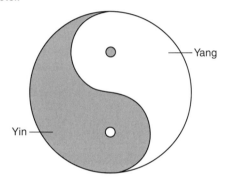

Figure 3.2   Yin and Yang – the Taoist symbol (From Cross 2001 *Acupressure and Reflextherapy*. Butterworth-Heinemann, with permission).

2. Yin and Yang are in a state of constant change. We cannot stop the passing of time.
3. Yin and Yang are opposites, but the essence of each is contained within the other because one will eventually turn into its opposite and can only exist because its opposite exists. Day turns into night.
4. Yin or Yang will predominate in any phenomena. We can say that the middle of the day is more Yang than the middle of the night.

Looking at the daily cycle of energy, we cannot just pick a time of day and say that it is Yin or Yang. We can only consider the quality of a time of day in relation to another time of day. Mid morning is Yin in relationship to midday but Yang in relationship to early morning.

The yearly (annual) movement of energy

Following on from the daily cycle of energy, we get the monthly and yearly changes of the seasons. Winter is the most Yin because it is the darkest and coldest season, and summer is therefore the most Yang. Yin is said to represent the element of water, expressing its qualities of coldness and wetness. Yang represents the opposite, the element of fire with its qualities of heat and dryness. The process of expansion produces heat and is Yang. When expansion is complete, there is less energy and therefore the process of moving back to Yin begins again.

The five phases theory, described below, provides a way of seeing the movements of energy as more than just the two extremes of summer, Yang, and winter, Yin, by attributing a different energy to each season.

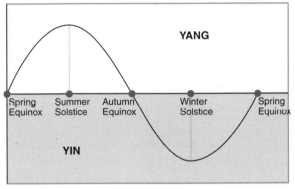

Figure 3.3   Yin and Yang as expressed in the annual cycle of the seasons.

After summer, the energy moves towards winter via autumn. It is about energy which is drawing in and contracting, and functions which are declining (Fig. 3.3). This is the element of metal which represents minerals and crystals.

After autumn, the energy declines still further into winter. This represents functions which have reached a maximal state of inward movement or rest, and are about to change the direction of their activity – water.

After winter comes spring, which represents the movement to Yang and active functions in a growing phase – wood.

After spring comes summer, which is about functions that have reached a maximal state of activity, Yang, and are about to move to Yin and begin a decline or resting period – fire.

The fifth phase is earth. Earth is said to be the buffer between the other phases – it is the basis for all change, representing the very earth itself.

Yin and Yang in the human body

If these principles are applied to the human body, we need to look at the body at its beginning – the embryo. In this curled-up form, the back is on the outside and the front of the body is on the inside. The inside relates to Yin as it is hidden and the outside, the back, relates to Yang (Fig. 3.4).

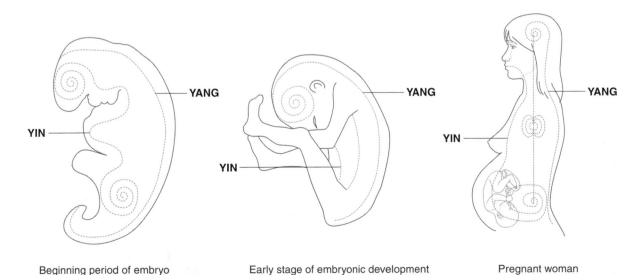

Beginning period of embryo   Early stage of embryonic development   Pregnant woman

Figure 3.4   Yin and Yang in the human body.

We can see immediately that Yang relates to the spinal cord and therefore the nervous system and the response of the body to outside influences. Yin represents the front of the body and links with the organs of the body and the digestive and reproductive systems. Yin relates more to material body and Yang relates to transforming processes in the body.

'Yang gives life, Yin makes it grow' (Yellow Emperor's Classic of Internal Medicine 1972).

From this understanding, we can draw up a whole list of phenomena which can be classified as representing the opposites of Yin and Yang. Yet it is important always to remember that they can only be classified as Yin and Yang because they

Table 3.2   Yin Yang correspondences

Categories	Yin	Yang
Earth – the macrocosm		
Sky	Moon	Sun
Time	Midnight	Midday
Season	Winter	Summer
Temperature	Cold	Hot
Humidity	Wetness	Dryness
Spectrum	Dark	Luminous
Realm	Hidden	Revealed
Solidity	Dense	Porous
Texture	Hard	Soft
Mass	Heavy	Light
Stages	Forming	Transforming
Movement	Descending, contracting	Ascending, expanding
Form	Material substance	Subtle influences
Human body – the microcosm		
Locale	Core, interior of body	Surface, exterior of body
	Front of body	Back of body
	Body	Head
	Below navel	Above navel
	Anterior medial surface of limbs	Posterior lateral surface of limbs
	Right side	Left side
Internal organs and meridians	Liver, Heart, Spleen, Lung, Kidney	Gall Bladder, Small Intestine, Stomach, Large Intestine, Bladder
Extraordinary vessels	Conception Vessel	Governing Vessel
Organ characteristics	Store essential and potential energy derived from substance	Process substances of the external environment
Constituents	Blood and metabolic fluids (Yin essence)	Ki and metabolic heat (Yang essence)
Processes	Build-up of tissue (anabolism)	Breakdown of tissue (catabolism)
Temperature	Coldness	Heat
Capacity	Weakness and depletion (empty – Kyo)	Strength and repletion (full – Jitsu)
Stages	Decline/death/gestation	Growth/birth/maturation
Dimension	Feelings and thoughts	Response and expression
Body type	Smaller, slender, sinewy, soft and dense	Larger, stronger, more tense, springy, muscular
	More limited capacity for food, work, interaction	Greater capacity for food and activity
	Avoids prolonged stress	Feels comfortable in stimulating environment, minimum capacity for rest
	Enjoys quiet	
	Tends to feel cold	Tends to feel warm
	Hypotensive	Hypertensive
	Delicate features	Coarse features
	Tends towards damp conditions	Tends towards dry conditions
Kind of illness	Illness develops gradually	Illness develops quickly
	Chronic conditions	Acute conditions
Physiological	Generation of blood, lymph, hormones, mucus, fat, collagen, perspiration	Process of circulation secretion, discharge peristalsis, pulsation metabolism, respiration
Reproduction	Egg	Sperm
Maternity	Pregnancy	Birth

have a relationship to each other – either as part of the universe or as part of the human body.

The expression of Yin and Yang in the body – the development of the first meridians

Yin and Yang flow in the body as different types of 'energy'. This energy expresses itself through the organs and physical structures of the body, and flows from them into the rest of the body through invisible energetic pathways, known as 'meridians'. 'Energy' and 'meridians' are really ways of looking at the inter-relationships between different parts of the whole. To a Western mind, these concepts can seem rather unreal, used as we are to thinking mostly about the physical body – what we can see. Modern science has tended to confirm that there are indeed pathways and connections. It is thought that the movements of energy which the Chinese were describing are linked with electromagnetic forces such as light, and the earth's and moon's magnetic and gravitational fields. These forces have been shown to act on each other and all living organisms to produce structural and functional effects and chronobiological rhythms. The initial energy which acts on the sperm and egg, resulting in the restructuring of the egg, can be said to relate to these gravitational forces (Brown & Park

1965). It is linked with the formation of the first meridians in the body. These are known as the extraordinary vessels of the Conception Vessel and Governing Vessel which represent the basic movement of Yin and Yang energy in the body.

The pathways of the Governing and Conception Vessels

One tangible way of looking at the embryonic development of these pathways is to see them as having developed from the two primitive germ layers of the endoderm (the Yin inner germ layer) and the ectoderm (the Yang outer germ layer). By day 14, a line of epiblast cells undergoes very rapid cell division, forming what is known as the primitive streak in the midline (Fig. 3.5). These cells form a groove and move inwards to spread between the two germ layers to form the middle layer of the mesoderm. At the cranial end of the streak is the small node called the primitive node which later becomes the neurenteric canal. Some mesodermal tissues proliferate from here to become the notochord; this establishes the development of the axial skeleton (bones of the head and spinal cord) and the neural plate of the ectoderm which gives rise to the primitive nervous system. This is the pathway of the Governing Vessel – the main meridian of the back of the body which governs the spine and brain. The endoderm

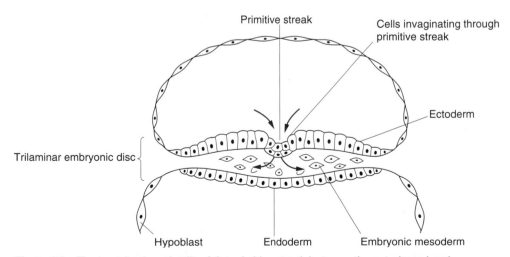

Figure 3.5 The invagination of cells of the primitive streak between the ectodermal and endodermal layers creates a trilaminar embryonic disc (From Fitzgerald & Fitzgerald 1994 *Human Embryology*. WB Saunders Company, with permission).

later forms the epithelial linings of the trachea, bronchi and lungs as well as the gastrointestinal tract. This is the pathway of the Conception Vessel – the main meridian of the front, or inside of the body, which governs the digestive system. The neurenteric canal itself allows communication between the neural tube of the ectoderm and the lining of the intestinal tract, the endoderm, which can help explain the relationship between the Conception Vessel and the Governing Vessel. The ectoderm and endoderm fuse at the oropharyngeal membrane (future mouth) and cloacal membrane (future anus) – which, interestingly, is where the Conception Vessel and Governing Vessel flow. Although they have two names, they are in fact branches of one pathway. These two meridians are known as the sea of Yin (Conception Vessel) and the sea of Yang (Governing Vessel) and are two of the most important meridians used when working with pregnant and labouring women.

The Chinese attributed various functions to these meridians. In order to understand this, we need to look a little more at what types of energy they identified as being in the body.

Different types of energy in the body

Although the body is seen as a whole, different types of energy flow within it. These different energies express themselves in both material and non-material forms. The energy most people have heard about is the energy known as Ki. This is the energy we draw on from day to day. It is what flows in the 12 main meridians, which develop from the initial endodermal/ectodermal circuit of the Conception Vessel and Governing Vessel as the fetus grows and the limb buds develop. The other most important form of energy is the Essence – which is the energy we draw upon as we grow, develop, reproduce and age. I will also briefly consider the energies of Blood and Shen.

Ki

Ki is the energy our body uses from day to day. It is ultimately regulated by the Conception Vessel and Governing Vessel, and flows through them and the 12 main meridians which transmit the energy of the organs into the rest of the body. It flows in the 12 meridians during a 24-h cycle and peaks in each meridian for a 2-h period during each day.

It is also known as Qi or Chi, and is the 'ki' in Reiki (universal energy) or the 'Chi' of Tai Chi or the 'Qi' of Qi Qung. Ki is considered to be the animating force behind life itself. There are different types of Ki in the human body although ultimately it is one energy which assumes different forms – all expressions of the Tao. Ki is invisible and is understood in terms of the effect it produces. It is about our ability to move our bodies, and governs the shape and activity of processes of organization and formation in the body. Physical and emotional activities are a manifestation of Ki. There are different types of Ki associated with particular actions or parts of the body: organ Ki, meridian Ki, nutritive Ki (associated with the Blood), protective Ki (responsible for resisting and combating external invasion of the body), Ki in the chest (ancestral Ki).

Ki is said to come from three different sources – original Ki, food Ki and air Ki. Original Ki is an energy which we inherit from our parents at the time of conception. This energy cannot be changed and we will see that it is part of our constitutional energy which is linked closely with another energy known as Essence. While in the womb, the fetus is nourished by the Ki of the mother. The baby starts producing its own Ki at the moment of birth when it begins to interact with the external environment. After birth, the baby's Lungs, Stomach and Spleen start functioning to produce Ki from food, drink and air.

This means that the quality of the food we eat is considered to be important. It is outside the scope of this book to cover diet but there are several good books on the Chinese approach to food. The best is by Paul Pitchford (Pitchford 1993).

Air Ki is formed not only by the way in which we breathe, but also by the way in which we move air/oxygen around the body. This explains the emphasis on exercise and breathing practices such as Tai Chi and Qi Qung in Eastern cultures. It is why stretches and passive movements of the body are part of shiatsu work and why shiatsu practitioners will emphasize the importance of correct breathing and appropriate exercise.

Suggestions will be made for this type of work through the book.

If our Ki is low, then, as it is renewed on a daily basis, changes in diet and exercise begin to have an effect quite quickly. It is interesting that the scientific approach to the body is now becoming more aware of how each cell is indeed made up of the air we breathe and the food we eat, and that this has an impact on the quality of our health.

We affect Ki through shiatsu by supporting the meridians that produce food and air Ki and by ensuring a smooth flow of Ki through the body in all meridians, organs and areas. Ki needs to flow in particular directions and sometimes it flows the wrong way so we need to move it. Sometimes we need to increase or decrease the flow of Ki in certain meridians or areas of the body. Sometimes we need to unblock it if it is stuck. This is why it is helpful to have some understanding of the functions of the meridians during pregnancy, birth and the postnatal period. In shiatsu our focus is to work with the concepts of Kyo and Jitsu, too little, or too much energy, and this will be explained in Section 3.

Essence (or Jing)

Essence is a crucial energy during pregnancy, birth and the postnatal period as it is the basis for reproduction and development. It is the substance that underlies all organic life and is the source of organic change. Essence is the deep or reserve energy that sustains us and is fluid-like, supportive and nutritive. It determines each person's basic constitutional make-up, strength, vitality, sexual, mental and defensive energies, as well as the material growth of bones, teeth, hair, brain development and sexual maturation. After puberty, it controls reproductive function and fertility. Essence is the energy that supports our longer-term growth and development, and is said to flow in 7-year cycles for women and 8-year cycles for men.

The Essence is stored in the Kidneys and is dependent on being nourished by them. Essence is a combination of what is known as 'pre-heaven Essence' and 'post-heaven Essence'. Pre-heaven Essence comes from the energy of our parents at the time of our conception and is fixed in quantity and quality. On one level, it is our genetic energy, but it is about more than the purely physical structure of the cells. It transmits emotional and spiritual patterns of energy as well and can be seen as our ancestral energy. It explains physical and behavioural patterns we see in families through the generations. 'Post-heaven Essence' is refined and extracted from food and fluids by Stomach and Spleen after we are born, and is the way we as individuals can influence our lives.

We draw on Essence through our life. It is said to peak in flow around ages 21–24, when we stop growing physically, and begins to weaken from 35 to 40. However, if our Essence is strong, even as we age, we can remain healthy in mind and body. It is more difficult to influence in adult life than Ki, but we can make the most of what we have by finding the balance between work/rest, diet and positive influences such as breathing exercises, T'ai Ji Quan and Qi Gong, shiatsu and acupuncture.

The mother's Essence, as well as her Ki, nourishes the embryo/fetus during pregnancy and supports the process of birth. With each child, the mother loses some of her Essence. This is not considered to be a problem because if her Essence is strong, it should be sufficient to support new life. If her Essence is weak, then problems may arise in pregnancy. The mother may feel very tired and suffer from all the complaints of pregnancy. It may cause development problems for the baby.

Essence circulates in the body through the circuit of the extraordinary vessels, ruled by the Governing Vessel and Conception Vessel; these therefore have a close relationship with the Kidneys, which store the Essence. It is interesting that modern science has discovered that the sexual organs, the testicles and ovaries, develop from the same tissue as the kidneys. In the embryo, these tissues, the nephrotomes, give rise to the nephric tubules in the developing urogenital ridges and traverse nearly the whole length of the embryo from head to tail. Although most of these tissues degenerate and are reabsorbed as the permanent kidneys develop, the communicative pathways of the tissues probably develop in these stages. It is fascinating that the Chinese were aware of this energetic connection from their observations and work with the body.

Essence is slower moving than Ki and flows deeper in the body. Essence is therefore more Yin and Ki more Yang. Unlike Ki, we can't increase the amount of Essence but we can still work to allow it to flow as well as it can in the body. The work is similar to working with Ki, but tends to involve more holding and deeper energetic connections because of its different nature. This will be explained in Section 3.

Shen

This is best translated as Spirit. It is the vitality behind Essence and Ki in the human body. Human consciousness indicates the presence of Shen. It is associated with the force of human personality, the ability to think, to discriminate, and choose appropriately. Its origin, like that of Essence, is created from the Shen of each parent. It does have a material aspect and is considered a Yang substance and as much a part of the body as any organ. The Heart is the most important organ that relates to Shen, and is said to nourish and anchor it through life including pregnancy and after birth.

Ki, Jing and Shen are known as 'the three treasures'.

Blood energy

This is not the same as the Western concept of blood. It moves through the blood vessels, but it also moves through the meridians. Just like, Ki, Shen and Essence, it is a form of energy which flows around the body. Unlike Ki, Shen and Essence, it is both a material substance as well as a process of generating, distributing and storing nutrients, nourishing the body. It originates through the transformation of food. Ki creates and moves the Blood and holds it in place. Blood in turn nourishes the organs which produce and regulate the Ki. Blood is Yin and Ki is Yang. Blood governs the tissue, the material form of the body.

There are several meridians/organs which relate to the Blood. Heart governs the Blood, by transforming food Ki into Blood and by governing circulation. Spleen makes the Blood by extracting Ki from food. Liver stores the Blood

and is its reservoir, sending out nourishment when it is needed. There is another extraordinary vessel (which I will discuss in the next section) which is said to be the origin of the Blood, the Penetrating Vessel. Blood therefore has a relationship with the Kidneys.

I will refer through the book to Blood as Blood energy, to help distinguish it from Western blood.

The pathways of energy – meridians and extraordinary vessels

The way that these different forms of energy travel around the body is along the pathways which we know as the meridians. Sometimes meridian is translated as 'channel'. These channels link the various organs, systems and substances in the body, forming an interconnecting network. They are considered to be branches of the source – the underlying unifying principle which the Chinese tried to describe through the Tao. The meridians have both internal and external pathways. Along the external pathways are important points on the skin known as the 'tsubos' which affect energy more profoundly. They link the inside of the body with the outside. It is at these places where the acupuncturist will insert needles. The shiatsu practitioner works with the tsubos but will also work with whole meridians, either using pressure or movements and stretches. By balancing the flow of energy in the meridians and points, the whole body will be more in harmony.

There are different types of meridians – many more than are represented by the 12 main meridians system with which you are probably most familiar.

'There is no part of the body, no kind of tissue, no single cell, that is not supplied by the channels' (Deadman et al 1998).

This book will examine the main meridians of importance in pregnancy, birth and the postnatal period. These include the 12 main meridians, responsible for the day-to-day circulation of energy from the main organs, four of the eight meridians known as the extraordinary vessels which have additional functions, and two other meridians which connect the Uterus.

The Western explanation of meridians

Research has put forward several ideas attempting to explain how shiatsu/acupuncture works from a Western perspective. Bensoussan (1991) draws together much of this research and argues that 'the primary mode of action of acupuncture' is the electromagnetic one (Yan et al 1986) which then influences physiological function such as tissue healing (Carley & Wainaple 1985, Wolcott et al 1969) and bone growth (Becker 1967). Bensoussan (1991) argues that 'neurological responses … occur as a result of changes in electromagnetic field patterns'.

Kiko Matsumoto and Stephen Birch (Matsumoto & Birch 1988) also examine Western explanations. They highlight the work of several leading researchers in Japan who have concluded that meridians lie in dermal connective tissues, specifically the superficial fascia (Motoyama 1980). Nagahama (1956) calls acupuncture 'connective tissue therapy'. James Oshman, in his book on connective tissue, highlights how this can then affect all systems in the body, 'All the great systems in the body – the circulation, the nervous system, the musculoskeletal system, the digestive tract, the various organs – are sheathed in connective tissue' (Oshman 1981).

This can help explain the wide-ranging effects of shiatsu and acupuncture. Connective tissue fibres are surrounded by interstitial fluids, which contain a vast array of chemicals, ionically charged particles, molecules and atoms, and they provide an interface with lymph and capillary systems; hence the cardiovascular effects that have been observed with acupressure (Manaka 1980). Application of pressure has been shown to generate small electric currents and tsubos have been found to coincide with areas on the body where there is lower electrical resistance (Nagahama 1956).

Another theory of action is that it is hormonally mediated (Bensoussan 1991). There has been shown to be a release of common neurotransmitters and hormones unique to each meridian, corresponding acupuncture point and internal organ after acupuncture, electrical stimulation, mechanical stimulation (including shiatsu), soft laser stimulation or Qi Gong. For example, encephalin, a neurotransmitter common to the gastrointestinal mucosa and the brain, is thought to play an important role in the control of pain by acupuncture. Connections have been found between each meridian and the corresponding internal organ areas in each side of the cerebral cortex (Omura 1989).

We will now consider in more detail the different functions of the extraordinary vessels and the 12 meridians, looking at both the physical and emotional aspects.

The functions of the Conception Vessel, Governing Vessel and the other extraordinary vessels

The extraordinary vessels are the first meridians to develop in the body from the primitive streak, and are considered to be the source of all energy flows and the reservoir of energy in the body. They are called 'vessels' to differentiate them from other meridians. 'Through embryological development and childhood they determine the growth of physical form' (Maciocia 1998). They provide the link between the Ki, our daily energy, and Essence, our constitutional energy. They represent a deeper level of treatment than work with the 12 meridians and are of particular importance in pregnancy. They have several functions:

To circulate and regulate Essence in the body. Essence cannot be increased, but its quality can be improved through its interaction with post-heaven Essence, which is largely determined by the Stomach and Spleen organ and meridian function. During pregnancy Essence needs to be sent to the baby as well as the mother.

To act as a reservoir for Ki and Blood energy in the body. They are the ultimate back-up system, rather like the reservoir for a city's water supply, with the 12 main meridians being the pipes and channels. When there is too much Ki in the system, they can draw it out and when there is not enough, they can send more out. During pregnancy, there are many changes in the flow of the mother's Ki – the extraordinary vessels help to regulate these changes.

To link the 12 main meridians. How the different extraordinary vessels do this will be discusssed under their specific descriptions.

To circulate defensive Ki. This protects the body from what the Chinese call 'exterior pathogenic factors'.

There are in total eight extraordinary vessels, but the Conception Vessel and the Governing Vessel are the only ones that have separate points and pathways from the other 12 meridians. The other six share their points with other meridians, which is an indication of the close relationship between them. Not all of them will be considered here; however, besides the Conception Vessel and Governing Vessel, there are two other important ones in pregnancy – the Penetrating Vessel

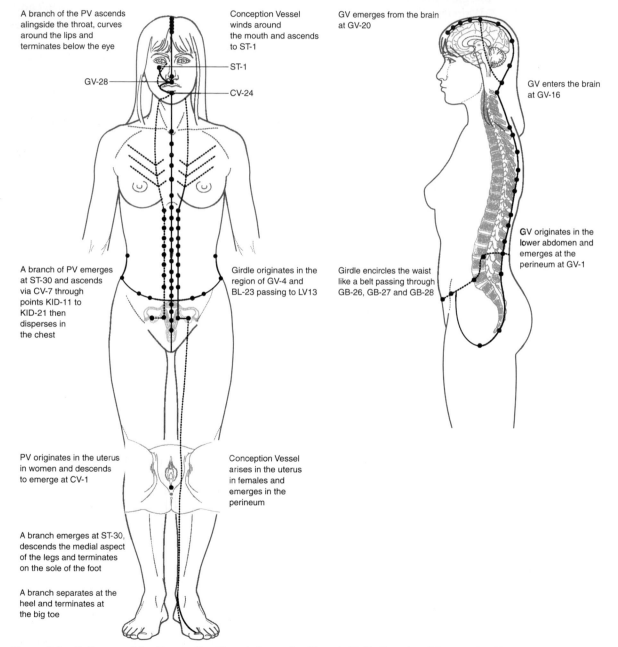

A branch of the PV ascends alingside the throat, curves around the lips and terminates below the eye

Conception Vessel winds around the mouth and ascends to ST-1

ST-1

GV-28

CV-24

GV emerges from the brain at GV-20

GV enters the brain at GV-16

A branch of PV emerges at ST-30 and ascends via CV-7 through points KID-11 to KID-21 then disperses in the chest

Girdle originates in the region of GV-4 and BL-23 passing to LV13

Girdle encircles the waist like a belt passing through GB-26, GB-27 and GB-28

GV originates in the lower abdomen and emerges at the perineum at GV-1

PV originates in the uterus in women and descends to emerge at CV-1

Conception Vessel arises in the uterus in females and emerges in the perineum

A branch emerges at ST-30, descends the medial aspect of the legs and terminates on the sole of the foot

A branch separates at the heel and terminates at the big toe

Figure 3.6 Pathways of the Conception Vessel, Governing Vessel, Girdle Vessel and Penetrating Vessel.

and the Girdle Vessel. The Penetrating Vessel is important because it is the third meridian to develop and is closely linked to the Conception Vessel and Governing Vessel. The Girdle Vessel is the only horizontal meridian in the body. As it encircles the pelvis, it is particularly important in pregnancy.

As we have already seen, the Governing Vessel and Conception Vessel are the first meridians to develop in the cell from the primitive streak and relate to the ectoderm and endoderm. The mesodermal layer of cells relates to the Penetrating Vessel.

These vessels originate from deep inside the human body, in the area between the Kidneys and the Uterus, which was considered by the Chinese to represent the source of all energy in the body. This point is known as the Ming Men. From here, they pass through the uterus in women, to emerge on the perineum and flow along their respective external pathways (Fig. 3.6). The Governing Vessel emerges on the perineum between the tip of the coccyx and the anus. It then flows right through the centre of the spine in the depressions between the spinous processes, continuing through the cervical vertebrae into the centre of the back of the head, over the top of the head and over the centre of the front of the face, to finish at a point on the upper lip and gum. The Conception Vessel emerges in the middle of the perineum and runs up the midline of the front of the body, through the centre of the throat, to finish at a point below the centre of the lower lip.

The Penetrating Vessel has a complex pathway and, unlike the Governing and Conception Vessels, it does not have its own independent points but shares points with some of the 12 meridians. It starts at the first point on the Conception Vessel on the centre of the perineum and then flows up to a point on the Stomach meridian (ST-30 – right on the top of the pubic bone two thumbwidths from the Conception Vessel on each side). This is an indication of the close relationship between Blood, Essence and the food we eat. It then flows up the centre of body in two pathways, each half a thumbwidth out from the midline in the abdomen and two thumbwidths from the midline in the chest, sharing its pathway with the Kidney meridian. This

indicates its close relationship with both the Kidney and Conception Vessel. It then flows up the throat, circles around the mouth and goes up to the forehead. A branch also goes up inside the spine, about the level of the fourth lumbar vertebra, thus following some of the Governing Vessel pathway.

Like all meridians, they have connections with more than just these external pathways. There is said to be another branch of the Conception Vessel which links up with the Governing Vessel at the top of the head, just in front of the crown at the point GV-20 – known as 'a thousand points of meeting'. All three meridians form one circuit linking the Kidneys, Heart and Brain. From a Western perspective, they can be said to represent the hypothalamus–pituitary–ovarian axis which is responsible for ovulation (Fig. 3.7). They relate via their connections with the other

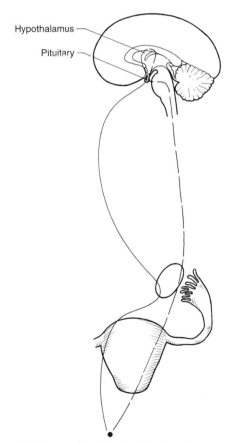

Figure 3.7   Governing and Directing Vessels as hypothalamus–pituitary–ovarian axis (From Maciocia 1998 *Obstetrics and Gynecology in Chinese Medicine*. Churchill Livingstone, with permission).

meridians to the rest of the body, including the arms and legs.

We can get an idea of the functions of meridians by looking at where they pass through the body; their functions relate closely to their origins in the different germ layers in the embryo. It is amazing how the Chinese understood this simply from observing how energy affected the body.

Governing Vessel – Sea of Yang

This develops from the ectoderm which relates to the neural tube, posterior pituitary and neural hormonal function, epidermis, surface of the body and the nervous system.

It strengthens and regulates Yang energy in the body and helps regulate the Ki of the six Yang meridians. As it runs through the spine, it is associated with any kind of spinal problem, whether structural or nervous. It relates to the nervous system, the neocortex and new brain functions. Emotionally, it is about someone's constitutional strength and their ability to interpret information.

Conception Vessel – Sea of Yin

This develops from the endoderm which relates to the gut tube, epithelium of the trachea, bronchi and lungs, the gastrointestinal tract, liver, pancreas, urinary bladder, pharynx, thyroid and parathyroids.

Matsumoto & Birch (1988) postulate that as the anterior pituitary is of epithelial ectodermal and gut endodermal origin, it is related to the Conception Vessel which can thus be said to govern metabolic hormonal function.

It strengthens and regulates all Yin energy in the body and helps regulate the Ki of the six Yin meridians. Passing through the front of the body, it relates to our digestive system and our ability to take in physical nourishment. It helps regulate breathing, the lungs and the ribs, and affects the abdominal muscles, especially the recti mucles. Of paramount importance for the reproductive system of women, it regulates menstruation, pregnancy, childbirth and menopause. Emotionally, it is about our ability to nourish ourselves, to be creative, our instinctive reactions and old brain functions.

Penetrating Vessel – Sea of Blood

This develops from the mesoderm which relates to the notochord, heart, blood vessels, blood, kidneys, spleen, connective tissues, fascia, muscles, cartilage and bones.

It strengthens and regulates Blood energy and is known as the Sea of Blood. It links the Stomach and Kidney meridians. In a way, it is the link between the Governing and Conception Vessels as it shares some of their pathways. Flowing closely to the Conception Vessel, it affects the abdominal muscles and, along with the Stomach, the breasts. It influences the supply and proper movement of Blood energy in the Uterus and has a crucial role in menstruation and during pregnancy in supplying Blood energy to the fetus. The Penetrating Vessel is about our ability to draw nourishment from the food we eat. It is often used if someone is feeling abdominal pain and distension, oppression in the chest and throat, a suffocating sensation, heat in the head, cold feet or anxiety including symptoms of fear and shock. It relates closely to the Heart and therefore has a key role in regulating all emotions.

Girdle Vessel

This is the only horizontal meridian in the body and binds the vertical paths of all 12 meridians as well as the Penetrating Vessel and Conception Vessel. It particularly connects the Spleen, Liver and Kidney meridians and passes through points associated with them. Like the Penetrating Vessel (and the other four extraordinary vessels which aren't discussed here), it does not have its own independent points. Its pathway is like a belt encircling the pelvis and it originates from the space between the Kidneys (GV-4) and passes under the rib cage, down the side of the body, over the anterior iliac spines to gather round the front of the body above the pubic bone. It affects both the bones and muscles of the pelvis, including the sacro-iliac joint, the symphysis pubis, internal and external obliques, transverse abdominal muscles as well as the deep and superficial muscles of the pelvic floor.

It guides and supports the Ki of the Uterus and the Essence. Ideally, it should be relaxed yet supportive. It is about our central physical support and how we emotionally anchor ourselves in the world.

The 12 meridians system

This system is responsible for the day-to-day circulation of Ki in the body. It comprises 12 main meridians. The three main meridians of back, front and side are shown in Fig. 3.8. They develop in the embryo after the main circuit of the extraordinary vessels as the limb buds develop. This is reflected in their main points being in the arms and legs as well as the torso. There is a difference here between the acupuncture system and the Zen meridian system developed by Masunaga (1977, 1987). In the traditional system, there are considered to be six meridians in the arms and six in the legs. Of these, three in the arms are Yin meridians and flow out from the body to the hand on the inside, the softer part of the arm. The other three are Yang meridians and flow from the hand to the body along the outside, the firmer part of the arm. The three Yin meridians in the arms are paired with three Yang meridians in the legs. The three Yang leg meridians flow from the top of the leg to the foot along the back, and the three Yin meridians flow from the foot up to the body. The direction of flow is the Yang meridians flowing down the body, if the person has the arms raised. The Yin flow is of meridians up the body.

Masunaga, in accordance with the Japanese view of the importance of the abdomen, the 'hara' (discussed in more detail later on pp. 74–75), realized through his work that there were other pathways of meridian flow. He found that the three Yin arm meridians had corresponding channels in the legs and vice versa, and that all meridians flowed through the hara. He developed an additional diagnostic system for assessing the energy in the meridians from specific areas related to each meridian in the hara. Many shiatsu schools today teach this extended meridian theory in addition to the traditional system. On the new meridians there are no tsubos. They are considered to be linking channels and to relate slightly more to the psychological rather than the physical aspects of the meridians. Masunaga applied his understanding of the meridians to exercise and has developed a series of meridian stretching exercises known as the Makkho exercises. It is these which you will find in Section 4. By practising this series of exercises, you will balance Ki in your body. Shiatsu, more than acupuncture, emphasizes the importance of preparation of the practitioner and for the client to take on aspects of their own self-healing. Exercise is a useful way of achieving this.

Box 3.1   Meridians summary box

There are different types of meridians:

- The eight extraordinary vessels. These are the first to develop in the embryo and are responsible for the flow of Essence and regulating Ki flow in the 12 meridians. Four of these vessels are covered in this book.
- The 12 meridians. These are the meridians with which you may be familiar. They form later in the embryo as the arms and legs develop and are responsible for the day-to-day circulation of Ki.
- Other meridians. There are many other meridians and linking channels. Two that are important in pregnancy, the Heart–Uterus and Kidney–Uterus, are discussed here.

Meridians influence the areas through which they pass. The Bladder meridian is the main Yang meridian of the back of the body and relates to the spine and the nervous system. It is closely related to the Governing Vessel. The Stomach is the main meridian at the front of the body and relates to the digestive system. It is closely related to the Conception and Penetrating Vessel.

In Section 3, I will not cover work with all the meridians, nor hara diagnosis, as this is a fairly complex skill. Midwives who wish to study shiatsu further may wish to undertake the 3-year shiatsu practitioner training which will include these skills. Much of the key shiatsu work in pregnancy, birth and the postnatal period can be achieved with knowledge of the most important meridians which will be described in Section 3. It is, however, useful to have an overall picture of all the meridians to understand how shiatsu works.

Functions of meridians

The 12 meridians are ordered in pairs. Each pair relates to one of the five elements and each partner within the pair expresses the Yin or Yang aspect of the element. Remember though, that

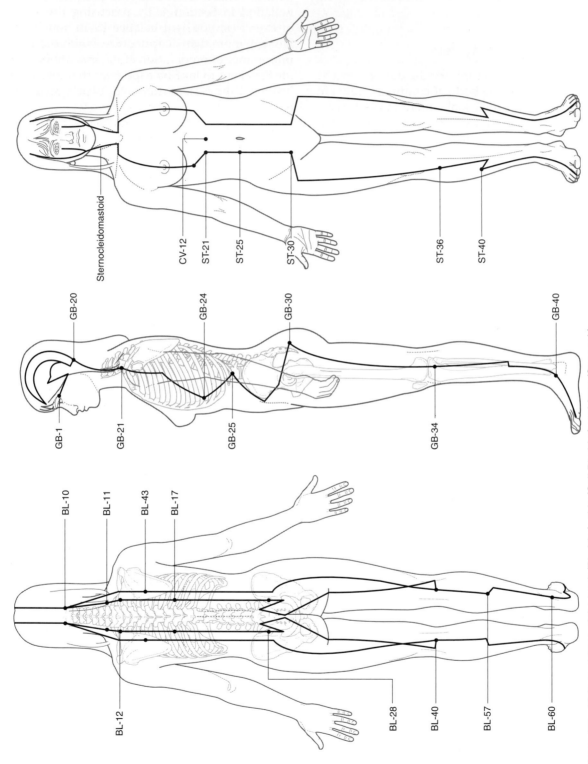

Figure 3.8 Main meridians of the back (Bladder), side (Gall Bladder) and front (Stomach).

there is Yin and Yang in everything and they are relative concepts. Like the three main extraordinary vessels, different meridians relate to the endoderm (Heart and Small Intestine, Kidney and Bladder), ectoderm (Lung and Large Intestine, Heart Protector and Triple Heater) and mesoderm (Stomach and Spleen, Liver and Gall Bladder). The 12 meridians are pathways transmitting the energy of the organ to the rest of the body. If you understand the function of the organ from a Western viewpoint you have a good starting point for understanding something about it from an Eastern viewpoint. However, Eastern thought defines organs/meridians by the functions associated with them unlike the Western view of defining from physical structure. This means they relate to more than the physical body and include emotional and spiritual aspects which are presented in Table 3.3.

For example, Lung is not simply the organ of the lungs but is about the whole process of taking in Air (which also is not seen as simply physically the molecules of air but a whole energy in itself). This process includes the skin, nose, trachea as well as the lungs. Energetically, it is about how we take anything in from the outside: this is where we get the correspondence of Lung to boundaries and its power being contraction – it is drawing energy in to the body. This is why the convention is to write the Eastern organ/meridian with a capital letter to differentiate it from the Western term. If you try to think of the whole cycle of energy of an organ, it is not too difficult to relate to how it is defined in Eastern thought.

Ideally, each person can express and relate to all five elements, indicating that energy is flowing well in their meridian system. What often happens though is that a person will relate much more to one or two elements and feel quite hostile to the energy of another element. They can become stuck in more negative aspects of that element. By balancing energy in the meridian system, people can begin to feel at home with the energy of all the elements and express their positive aspects. The elements and organs interact with each other, and many different theories have evolved to explain the complex relationships between them all. Some of these relationships will be discussed here, but not in great detail.

By understanding the energy of each element it is not actually that difficult to see how it is going to relate to other elements. For example, as you would expect, water is said to control fire i.e. it puts it out. What is most important is to balance the two most out-of-balance elements. In Section 3 we will learn how to do this appropriately – either by bringing more energy to one where there is not enough or taking energy away from one where there is too much.

Lung and Large Intestine – metal element

Energetic pattern – exchange and elimination.

Metal in nature   In a way, this is the most difficult element to understand. As metal is the movement from Yin to Yang, this energy is considered to be about contraction, things drawing in, like crystals forming. It relates both to the air and to the structure of the earth, the rocks, crystals, minerals. The Yin aspect of air is stillness and calm. The Yang aspect is wind, active movement of air. In minerals, the Yin aspect is related to a formed crystal, which may be cold. Yang is the molten lava, bubbling away.

Lung   The Yin aspect is about the in-breath and the intake of Ki energy in the form of air which is fundamental to life. The Yang aspect is the out-breath and elimination of unwanted gases. It governs Ki and disperses and spreads defensive Ki all over the body. It is linked with the immune system and is the first line of the immune response. It expresses itself in the skin. Lung energy needs to move down to the Large Intestine to help with defecation.

Large Intestine   It helps the function of Lung. It receives the energies of food and drink from the Small Intestine. Together they are seen as taking in what we need and then letting go of the waste – both physically and emotionally.

Personality type   They are about how we define and value our self in the world. They are often quite clear, incisive thinkers but find it more difficult to express emotions and often hold on to them, which is where we get the correspondence of grief.

Stomach and Spleen – earth element

Energetic pattern – ingestion and digestion.

Table 3.3 Chart of the main meridian correspondences

Element	Wood	Fire	Earth	Metal	Water
Yin organ/meridian	Liver	Heart and Heart Protector	Spleen	Lungs	Kidney
Yang organ/meridian	Gall Bladder	Small Intestine and Triple Heater	Stomach	Large Intestine	Bladder
Season	Spring	Summer	Transition between seasons – the centre	Autumn	Winter
Climate	Windy	Hot	Damp	Dry	Cold
Colour	Green	Red, purple	Yellow/orange	White	Black/blue
Time of peak flow	11 pm–3 am	11am–3pm 7pm–11pm	7–11am	3–7am	3–7pm
Tissue	Tendons/ligaments	Blood vessels	Flesh/muscles	Skin	Bones, head hair
Orifice	Eyes	Tongue	Mouth	Nose	Ears
Sense organ	Eyes	Tongue	Mouth	Nose	Inner ear
Fluid secretion	Tears	Perspiration	Saliva – mouth	Mucous	Saliva in mouth
Physical expression	Nails, hands, feet	Complexion	Flesh	Skin and body hair	Bones and bone marrow, head hair
Taste	Sour	Bitter	Sweet	Pungent	Salty
Human sound	Shouting	Laughing	Singing	Weeping	Groaning
Emotion	Anger – can feel frustrated if not in control; can become resentful	Joy – but this can be an over joyous, over excitable state; can turn into bitterness	Sympathy/thinking – can concentrate too much on detail and end up going round in circles; can turn to disgust and self pity	Grief – if we do not let go we hold on and grieve; can become disdainful	Fear – can turn to paranoia
Power	Expansion Control	Fusion	Moderation	Contraction	Consolidation
Desires	Purpose	Fulfilment	Connectedness	Order	Truth
Virtues	Fervour Discernment	Charisma Insight	Loyalty Integrity	Righteousness Balance	Honesty Wisdom
Life expression	Spiritual faculties	Spirit	Ideas/opinions	Animal spirit	Will power and ambition
Talent	Initiative	Communication	Negotiation	Discrimination	Imagination
Existential issue	Goals – what to do? strategy – how to do it	Dimension – how broad is my scope?	Orientation – what's my role? where am I?	Boundaries – what I am and am not	Origins/destiny – what is my past, what is my future?

Earth in nature   Earth is the soil, the very basis for nourishing all life forms. The Yin aspects are the wet, damp, fertile earth. The Yang aspects are dry and arid, hot earth, scorched earth. Earth is the centre of the elements and considered to be the balance between Yin and Yang. This is where we get the aspects of stability, the home, the centre linked with earth.

Spleen   Spleen makes Ki and Blood from the energy of food. It controls the Blood, holds it in the vessels and breaks down red blood cells. It raises energy up, especially along the midline of the body. It is about transportation and transformation. It controls the initial phase of separation of food energy into pure and impure, and all phases of body fluid production – especially gastric bile, secretions for the small intestine and reproductive hormones linked to the breast and ovaries. Spleen is affected by damp, as it gives it more fluids to process. It is sometimes known as Spleen/Pancreas as it encompasses the functions of the Western pancreas and is about sugar regulation in the body.

Stomach   This takes in food and transforms it ready for the Spleen to separate and extract the refined essence. It sends energy down to the Small Intestine. It is the main meridian of the front of the body.

Personality type   This is the centre of all the elements and is the dependable type, the quiet centre where people feel at home. The person's relationship with food is often an issue. They tend to like sweet foods, overeat and often express themselves through cooking and caring for others.

Heart and Small Intestine – fire element

Energetic pattern – conversion and integration.

Fire in nature   The Yin aspect is the quiet, glowing fire contained in a heart or the candle slowly burning – still but shining light. The Yang aspect is the raging fire, like a bush fire, burning everything down and becoming uncontrolled. Fire is the most Yang of all the elements and tends to burn things up and be all-consuming. When it gets out of hand, it tends to flow up the body.

Heart   Heart rules the Blood, controls the blood vessels, manifests in the complexion, houses the Mind (Shen), opens into the tongue and controls sweat. Heart loathes heat. As the Shen expresses

the whole emotional, mental and spiritual aspects including consciousness, memory, thinking and sleep, Heart is said to be the overall ruler of the emotions. It is about the capacity to form relationships with others and it controls speech.

Small Intestine   This may seem an odd meridian to pair with the heart, but in fact it has been shown that the heart in the embryo develops from the same layer of tissues as the Small Intestine. Small Intestine is considered to be like the First Minister to the Heart, which was the Emperor. Not many people would get to see the Emperor himself, but the First Minister would pass their messages on to the Heart and transmit the will of the heart to the people. In this way, the Small Intestine is said to have an influence on mental clarity and judgement. It is about the final stages of the digestion of food – separating the pure from the impure. In times of shock it sends blood out to where it is needed and draws in from the extremities.

Personality type   Typically, they are very active and excitable people, who like to be the centre of attention and for other people to notice them. Relationships are extremely important to them and they can find it difficult to be on their own. Their moods can go up and down quite easily.

Triple Heater and Heart Protector – supplemental fire element

Energetic pattern – circulation and protection.

Supplemental fire   These are also related to fire and represent a quieter version of fire energy.

Triple Heater – three burners   The Triple burner is fairly complex to understand as it does not relate to any definable organ but to what are known as the three burning spaces. It is however considered to be one of the most important meridians as it links together the Kidney, the Governing and Conception Vessels and the 12 meridians and organs. The three burners are spaces related to areas in the body:

1. The upper burner is in the centre of the sternum and relates to Lung and Heart Protector (functions of exchange of energy) and the thymus.
2. The middle burner is the area below the xiphoid process (the piece of cartilage at the lower

end of the sternum) and above the navel, and relates to Spleen and Stomach and functions of digestion.

3. The lower burner is in the area below the navel and above the pubic bone, and relates to Bladder and Kidney and processes of elimination of energy, as well as the lacteal ducts (lymphatic capillaries in the walls of the small intestine) and the cisterna chyli (thoracic duct in the abdomen which serves as a storage area for lymph moving back to its point of entry in the venous system).

Extending through the body from back to front, the burners link the energy of the Governing Vessel and Conception Vessel, sharing points with them. The Three Burner energy is said to arise at the area of moving Ki between the Kidneys, Ming Men, from where the extraordinary vessels also arise. It is the messenger of the source Ki, the basic energy in the body, and sends energy to some important points on meridians. It regulates fluids and lymph, rules the fascia and has important immune functions.

Heart Protector   This has a close relationship with Heart and is rather like the pericardium. It protects the heart physically, relating to blood vessels and lymph ducts as well as emotionally.

Bladder and Kidncy – water element

Energetic pattern – supplying vital energy and purifying body fluids.

Water in nature   Water is essential for life and represents the basic life force and survival instinct. Yin aspects relate to still water which could turn into a stagnant pond. Yang aspects relate to a river flowing on and on, the power of water to create dramatic changes. This is the most Yin of the elements and therefore tends to stillness and to depletion.

Kidney   In Chinese terms, this element relates to water function in the body. It governs the flow of fluids in the body – both those which have a physical base such as blood, lymphatic, endocrine, urinary, perspiration, saliva, tears, sexual secretions, as well as those with an emotional base such as thoughts, emotions and feelings. It includes the adrenals and therefore the 'fight or flight' response and is linked with the endocrine system.

The Kidneys relate to urination and to the purification of the Blood. They are known as the 'Gateway to the Stomach' as they assist the function of the Stomach organ. Kidney stores the Essence which governs birth, growth, reproduction and development.

Bladder   It removes water by the transformation of Ki. It relates to the midbrain and connects the Kidney hormone system with the pituitary gland. It is connected to the autonomic nervous, reproductive and urinary systems and is responsible for the elimination of urine – the final product of body liquid purification. It affects the spine as it passes through the erectae spinae muscles and can be said to be both our physical and emotional support/back-up system.

Together, Kidney and Bladder regulate fluids in the body, nourish the brain and influence short-term memory. Essence produces Marrow, which is not bone marrow in the Western sense, but a substance that is the common matrix of bones, bone marrow, brain and spinal cord. Bladder and the Masunaga extended Kidney meridian are the main meridians of the back of the body.

Personality type   They are often very driven people. Like water which doesn't know when to stop, they can be ready to get up and go at a moment's instance. This reflects the link with the adrenal system. They are often hard working and ambitious. In expressing the more Yin aspects of water, they can also be psychic and tune in to many different types of energies. Like water, they can be very adaptable and can assume different types of personality depending on the situation.

Liver and Gall Bladder – wood element

Energetic pattern – storage and distribution.

Wood in nature   Wood is tree energy – vital and growing upwards but also with its roots firmly planted in the earth. It is about the movement towards the Yang energy of fire, but still retains its links with the earth. Healthy wood energy is both grounded and expansive at the same time. The Yin aspects are to do with the rooted qualities and attraction to moisture and the earth. The Yang is about the upward growth of the branches. The tendency can be for the wood not to take the nourishment from the earth and become dry and brittle, unable to change or move.

Liver Liver stores Blood energy; it has an important function in menstruation and in regulating the volume of Blood in the body. When the body is at rest Blood flows to the Liver; when it is active it flows out to the muscles. This means that it is responsible for ensuring a smooth flow of Ki. It is about the storage and distribution of energy.

Gall Bladder It stores and excretes bile and unlike the other Yang organs doesn't communicate with the outside world. It is the only Yang organ to store a clean fluid. It controls judgement and the sinews.

They are the main meridians of the side of the body.

Personality type In balance, they are a spiritually aware person, growing in an expansive yet grounded way. Typically they like to be in control, like a general in charge of armies, having an overview of the situation and delegating where appropriate. They can get stuck when they don't delegate. If wood energy is not strong they can suffer from being indecisive. If wood types don't express their emotions, they can build up in the body as anger and frustration, exploding on occasion. If wood energy is too strong, then they may always seem to talk in a loud voice.

The Uterus and its meridians

It is worth considering the Uterus and its meridians, even though they do not form part of the main organ/meridian system, because of their importance in the antenatal, intrapartum and postnatal periods. The Uterus is classed as one of the Six Extraordinary Yang Organs, the others being the Brain, Bones, Marrow, Gall Bladder and Blood Vessels. In shiatsu, the Uterus is called the Bao Gong (literally 'Palace of the Child') and it includes the fallopian tubes and the ovaries. It can be considered to be linked with the earth element as it is in the centre of the body and provides the 'soil' for the seed of the fertilized egg to implant.

Both the Conception and Penetrating Vessels originate from the Kidney, flow through the Uterus and help it to regulate menstruation, conception and pregnancy. The Conception Vessel provides Ki and the Penetrating Vessel provides Blood energy to the Uterus.

Heart–Uterus meridian (Bao mai) There is a direct connection between the Heart and the Uterus via this meridian. It nourishes the Uterus with Blood sent down from the Heart. It provides a link between fire and earth elements. There can be disturbance in this meridian if there is stress on the mother's Heart (for example, through mental agitation or emotional frustration) which will affect the baby in the womb emotionally.

The Kidney–Uterus channel (Bao luo) There is a channel which connects the Kidneys with the Uterus. This nourishes the uterus with Essence. It provides a link between the water and earth elements. Overwork and exhaustion, as well as fertility treatment which overstimulates the Essence, all deplete its energy.

Summary

We have now discussed the key concepts of Chinese medicine. In the next chapter, we will look at how Chinese medicine can be used to explain the energy patterns in the different phases of pregnancy, birth and the postnatal period.

Reflect on the following questions:

- Which element do you feel most at home with?
- Which element do you not relate to?
- Think of women in your care and see if you can begin to look at some of them in the light of how they express or don't express the energy of the different elements

REFERENCES

Becker R O 1967 Electrical control of growth processes. Medical Times 95:657–669

Bensoussan A 1991 The vital meridian. Churchill Livingstone, Edinburgh

Brown F A Jr, Park Y H 1965 Phase shifting a lunar rhythm in Planarians by altering the horizontal magnetic vector. Biology Bulletin 129(1):79

Carley P J, Wainaple S F 1985 Electrotherapy for acceleration of wound healing: low intensity direct current. Archives of Physical Medicine and Rehabilitation 66:443–446

Cho Z H, Whang E K et al 2000 Functional magnetic resonance in the investigation of acupuncture. In: Stux G, Hammerschlag R (eds) Clinical acupunture, scientific basis. Springer, Berlin

Cross J R 2001 Acupressure and reflextherapy. Butterworth-Heinemann, London

Deadman P, Al-Khafaji M, Baker K 1988 Manual of acupuncture. Journal of Chinese Medicine Publications, Hove

Fitzgerald M J T, Fitzgerald M 1994 Human embryology. Baillière Tindall, Edinburgh

Fukada E, Yasuda I 1957 On the piezoelectric effect of bone. Journal of the Physical Society of Japan 12:149–154

Health Statisitics Office 2000 Report on public health administration and services year 2000, statistics on health administration and services. Vital and Health Statistics Division, Statistics and Information Department, Ministers Secretariat, Ministry of Health, Labour and Welfare, Japan

Kushi M 1977 The book of macrobiotics. Japan Publications, Tokyo, p 11

Maciocia G 1989 The foundations of Chinese medicine. Churchill Livingstone, Edinburgh

Maciocia G 1998 Obstetrics and gynaecology in Chinese medicine. Churchill Livingstone, Edinburgh

Manaka Y 1980 Shinkyu no Riron to Kangaekata [thoughts and theory of acupuncture and moxibustion], 2nd edn. Sogen Igaku Sha, Osaka, Japan

Masunaga S 1977 Zen shiatsu. Japan Publications, Tokyo

Masunaga S 1987 Zen imagery exercises. Japan Publications, Tokyo

Maternal and Child Health Statistics of Japan 2001 Live birth by place of birth, urban and rural, 1950–2000. Maternal and Child Health Division, Equal Employment, Child and Families Bureau, Ministry of Health, Labour and Welfare, Japan, p 45

Matsumoto K, Birch S 1988 Hara diagnosis, reflections on the sea. Paradigm Publications, Brookline, Massachusetts, USA

Motoyama H 1980 Electrophysiological and preliminary biochemical studies of skin properties in relation to the acupuncture meridian. International Association for Religion and Parapsychology, Tokyo

Nagahama Y 1956 Skinkyu no Igaku [Western studies of acupuncture and moxibustion]. Sogen Sha, Osaka, Japan

Ohashi W 1977 Do it yourself shiatsu. Unwin Paperbacks, London

Omura Y 1989 Acupuncture and electrotherapeutics research. Heart Disease Research Foundation 14(2):155–186

Oshman J 1981 The connective tissue and myofascial systems. Rolfing '81, Aspen Research Institute, Los Angeles

Pitchford P 1993 Healing with whole foods, oriental traditions and modern nutrition. North Atlantic Books, Berkeley, California, USA

Takahashi K 1996 Acupressure by nurse midwives in Japan. In: The art and science of midwifery gives birth to a better future. Proceedings of the International Confederation of Midwives 24th Triennial Congress, 26–31 May 1996, Oslo. International Confederation of Midwives, London, pp 435–439

Tempaku T 1915 Shiatsu ryoho. Japan

Wolcott L E, Wheeler P C, Hardwicke H M, Rowleg B A 1969 Accelerated healing of skin ulcers by electrotherapy; preliminary clinical results. Southern Medical Journal 62:795–801

Yan J, Yi S X, Wang L H et al 1986 An observation of muscular electricity of 'propagated sensation along the meridian'. Second National Symposium of Acupuncture and Moxibustion and Acupuncture Anaesthesia, Beijing, paper no 311

Yellow Emperor's classic of internal medicine – simple questions. People's Health Publishing House, Beijing. First published c. 100 BC. Translated by Ilza Veith 1949, University of California Press Ltd, Berkeley, CA, USA, first paperback edition 1972

4

The antenatal, intrapartum and postnatal periods from a shiatsu perspective

Introduction

The focus in Chinese medicine is not in trying to classify illness. Instead it looks at the whole person who has a tendency to develop certain types of conditions. The aim is to support a healthy body in its natural functions and rhythms, rather like tending a garden, not in waiting for an energetic imbalance to develop into illness. Indeed, some Chinese doctors were paid when the patient was well, not when they were sick – true preventative medicine. This approach is extremely well suited to pregnancy, which, although not a time of illness, is a time when many physical, emotional and spiritual demands are placed on the body.

Main energy changes and patterns during pregnancy for the mother

At the moment of conception, Yang is the sperm that provides the spark of energy to begin the process of transforming the Yin egg into the embryo/fetus and baby. Pregnancy is about the development of a material being and takes place in the watery environment of the womb – Yin energy in relation to conception and birth. To support this growth, there is a change in the flow of energies in the mother's body. The fetus must receive Essence (Jing) from the mother's Kidneys as well as her Ki and Blood energy. The mother needs to have enough of these energies to nourish the baby and they need to be able to flow freely to the Uterus. The Chinese understood that the cessation of menstruation meant that more

Blood energy was available, mirroring what we know physiologically about the maternal increase in blood volume. Blood and body fluids are part of Yin fluids. For all these reasons, pregnancy is considered to be a Yin state. Of course there are Yang aspects to pregnancy. The absence of periods leads to an accumulation of fire heat in the body and heat needs to be supplied to the fetus. This is how the Chinese viewed the rise in core body temperature in pregnancy.

In pregnancy, energetically women do tend to want to move inside themselves, mirroring the movement of Yin energy. Their bodies' focus is on the growing baby. In traditional Japan, indeed in many pre-industrial societies, pregnancy was a time when women were encouraged to take more care of themselves. They would follow special diets and lifestyle changes (Goldsmith 1984). Massage and shiatsu were often used to support them. Although women would still work, the work was in the home or community which was part of their support system and would adapt to their changing needs. In our culture, women tend to be working in environments that regard their pregnant state as something to be ignored, if anything rather a nuisance. Women's energy is focused away from their bodies' needs, into a more Yang sphere of activity. This can sometimes create tension, depending on how much space the woman has to balance the demands of her job with the demands of her body and her baby.

We could say that it is even more important for a woman working outside the home to receive regular shiatsu and massage to help her slow down and allow energy to flow to her baby. My own clinical observations indicate that women who work too hard tend to have small babies or even develop pre-eclampsia. From a shiatsu viewpoint, we can say that it is their bodies' energy expressing an imbalance, usually to do with Kidney and Liver energy, expressing very tangibly that it can't do everything.

We can, on a simple level, classify people into two main types – the Yin type and the Yang type. The Yin person who becomes pregnant would probably be more drawn to wanting to slow down. It is possible that she already has a quieter kind of work which allows plenty of time for self-reflection. She might work on her own, or at least have a job that gives her freedom to work at her own pace. Yin-type people do not tend to perform well under pressure. When she is pregnant, she may find she wants to slow down even more, and may find ways of cutting back her hours and having plenty of maternity leave. Her energy is more in tune with the Yin inward-looking aspect of pregnancy. If she doesn't find ways of slowing down, she is likely to get quite ill – coping with a job and with pregnancy can be too much of a strain on her body. She could be the type who seems drained by her pregnancy and gets tired very easily. Her type of illness would be of the more chronic type – continued levels of tiredness, anaemia, or persistent backache.

On the other hand, the Yang person would be involved in a more active job, often working a lot with other people and performing to deadlines. If in her pregnancy she can slow down a little and take time for quieter moments with herself and her baby, she may well find she is able to still remain quite active and not feel too tired. If, however, she continues to live life at the same pace, ignoring her body's messages to slow down, she may find that she becomes resentful of the baby and can even become quite ill with the pregnancy. Her type of illness would tend to be more extreme and dramatic – pre-eclampsia, hypertension or going into labour early.

Although the baby is drawing on the mother's energies, pregnancy needn't necessarily weaken a woman as it depends on how good her energy was before she conceived and how she looks after herself during the pregnancy. However, if any of her energies are insufficient, problems may arise with the growth and development of the fetus and the successful completion of gestation.

The main focus therefore of work in pregnancy is to maintain the best, most balanced production and flow of Ki, Blood energy and Essence. If any of these fail to flow well, then both the mother and the baby will be affected.

Questions

From your understanding of energy flows in Chinese medicine, which meridians do you think you will need to work to influence Ki, Blood energy and Essence? Look back to pages 36–38 to remind yourself.

Flow and production of Essence

This relates mostly to the energy of the Kidneys, which store the Essence, and the extraordinary vessels of the Governing Vessel, Conception Vessel, Penetrating Vessel and Girdle Vessel which circulate the Essence. It relates to the Kidney–Uterus meridian which is responsible for the flow of Essence to the Uterus. Constitutional weakness of Kidney Essence, which may be a result of the woman's mother being old when conceiving her, or the parents' having a poor constitution or poor long-term physical or psychological health at the time of conception, may lead to infertility or miscarriage.

It is not possible to increase the amount of Essence that someone has, but it is possible to balance how it is moved around the body through working these meridians, especially in making sure that it gets to the baby as well as the mother. The quality of Essence is affected by its interaction with the energy of food, processed mainly by Stomach and Spleen. Shiatsu work with these meridians will be important, as will attention to proper diet and physical nourishment.

Flow and production of Ki

The Conception Vessel and Governing Vessel are the regulators of Yin and Yang Ki in the body, especially in times of change. In the first trimester, there are big changes in Ki flow in the body as Ki needs to be directed to the uterus to nourish the placenta and the baby. Ultimately, all the 12 meridians are affected in different ways as they circulate different types of Ki, all of which are important for the baby.

It is possible to assess the woman's posture and see physically where the flow of energy is flowing or blocked at different stages of the pregnancy. As the baby grows, so the abdomen distends and pressure is put on the abdominal organs and meridians, especially Heart–Uterus, Penetrating Vessel and Conception Vessel. The development of the linea negra indicates some women's response to the changes in the Conception Vessel. Both Ki and body fluids find it more difficult to flow up and down the body during pregnancy. Energy is said to be blocked specifically

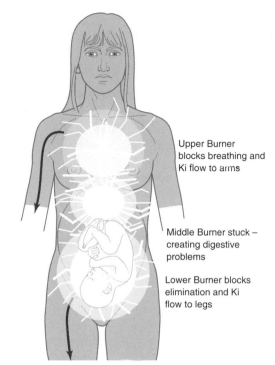

Upper Burner blocks breathing and Ki flow to arms

Middle Burner stuck – creating digestive problems

Lower Burner blocks elimination and Ki flow to legs

Figure 4.1 Ki flows, showing how the baby in the lower burner blocks the flow of energy to the mother's arms and legs.

in the Three Burners – the baby prevents energy from moving between them, and the energy tends to get stuck in the middle burner, affecting digestion. This blocks energy flow into the upper burner and the arms and chest, affecting breathing. It blocks the flow of energy in the lower burner affecting Bladder and Kidney and the flow of energy down to the mother's legs (Fig. 4.1).

The increasing weight of the baby tends to place strain on the back, creating lordosis and affecting the flow of the Governing Vessel.

Flow and production of Blood energy

The Penetrating Vessel is the Sea of Blood. Other important meridians are the Spleen, which produces the Blood, the Liver, which stores the Blood, and the Heart, which rules the Blood. Heart–Uterus sends Blood and emotional energy to the Uterus. Menstrual blood is not seen as Blood energy in Chinese terms, but as a precious fluid, which is no longer lost each month and nourishes the pregnant body in a form of Essence.

After conception, some Blood energy is gradually transformed to Milk energy, in preparation for breastfeeding. It transfers its location from the lower to the upper burner. This contributes to morning sickness, the general feeling of heat rising in the upper body and distension of the breasts.

Now we will consider in more detail the effects on the specific meridians.

Governing, Conception and Penetrating Vessels – regulators of many changes

We could say, on one level, that it is these vessels that provide the link between the changes in flow and production of Essence and Ki (which they all regulate) and Blood energy, which the Penetrating Vessel regulates. They are the basis for follicle maturation, ovulation and corpus luteum development. If any of these are not functioning well, then this can lead to problems both for the mother and the baby.

Penetrating Vessel

In the first trimester, it needs to send increased Blood energy to the Uterus to nourish the development of the blastocyte, into embryo and fetus, and to establish the placenta and amniotic sac. Until the placenta is established, there is nowhere for this energy to be physically held and so it tends to flow back up the mother's chest creating feelings of suffocation and heat in her upper body, sometimes causing feelings of anxiety. As the Kidney and Penetrating Vessel are closely linked, this rising Penetrating Vessel energy may drain her Kidney energy and lead to it becoming depleted in the lower abdomen and back. This often leads to feelings of tiredness and weakness in these areas.

Stomach energy works with the Penetrating Vessel. It needs to flow down to keep the Penetrating Vessel anchored in the lower abdomen. If the Stomach is weak and fails to do this, the upward movement of the Penetrating Vessel will be aggravated, creating feelings of nausea and sickness. Other meridians, such as the Liver, can also flow upwards causing more extreme vomiting and sickness.

Once the placenta is established, the Penetrating Vessel energy tends to settle down again in the lower abdomen and this is why morning sickness usually declines at the end of the first trimester, unless the patterns of weak Stomach and upward flowing Liver are extreme, in which case the result may be hyperemesis. In the second trimester, the mother can have a blooming complexion, feel her Blood energy is flowing well and be emotionally quite contented and settled. By the end of the third trimester, the baby is drawing more and more on the Penetrating Vessel energy to support its rapid weight gain and this is why the mother can begin to feel more tired again and tend towards anaemia. She may begin to feel anxious, especially with the impending birth, and feel weakness in the lower back.

Case study 4.1   Helen – a midwife shiatsu practitioner from New Zealand

A midwife and part-time yoga teacher to pregnant women, I completed my shiatsu training in 1999. I particularly find a deeper connection between myself and my client when using the Conception Vessel and Penetrating Vessel. One of my clients describes … 'I go to my shiatsu session feeling fragmented, and come away feeling as if everything has been put back together. Shiatsu has really helped me concentrate on the baby and my changing body and to slow down. The focus on the breath is peaceful. The touch, an intention that is for me and the baby, and the benefits that shiatsu gives with the gentle pooling of energy needed for pregnancy, provides the deepest relaxation and contentment'.

Shiatsu has also brought new meaning to my yoga teaching as I can use exercises with more awareness that stimulate specific meridians. I work in the delivery suite of my local maternity hospital and feel privileged to be in the right place to help consenting women, using techniques that can reduce pain and promote a more efficient and spontaneous labour and birth.

Conception Vessel

This provides Yin energy to the uterus, fetus and placenta. With so much Yin energy focused on the baby, the mother may find she lacks enough for herself. She may feel tired and exhausted, and have problems with breathing and digestion. This links closely to the pattern described of energy not moving in the chest and the three burners. Along with Stomach, it governs the recti muscles and needs to be strong to minimize their natural softening and give support to the abdomen. A lot of the mother's creative energy is focused on creating new life, she may find her focus of creativity switches to activities focused on her new baby such as nest-building.

Governing Vessel

This needs to provide Yang energy to the fetus, often in the form of heat and warmth. It is related closely to the spine through which it flows and so is responsible for the basic structural support of the body. Many women suffer from backaches and lack of Yang energy in pregnancy. Forgetfulness and a lack of focus, especially in responding to external stimuli, are a sign of weakened energy. The mother may find it hard to keep up with demands unrelated to her focus on the baby.

Effects on the Girdle Vessel, Heart–Uterus and Kidney–Uterus

Girdle Vessel

This energy needs to support the baby in the uterus, as well as the uterus in the abdomen and the pelvis, with Essence and Ki. Along with the Conception Vessel, it supports the abdominal muscles, especially the internal and external obliques. Its energy is like that of a girdle and if it is not strong can become slack – this can be a cause of miscarriage. Slack or weak energy can also lead to problems with supporting the muscles, ligaments and joints of the pelvis such as the sacro-iliac and the symphysis pubis. It may not hold the baby in a good position, thus letting the baby 'fall out' into the transverse or oblique position. On the other hand, the energy may be too strong such that the girdle feels too tight, the baby may be held in an unfavourable position such as breech, or the mother may find it difficult to give birth and let the baby be born.

It links Spleen, Liver and Kidney energies (see later in this chapter).

Box 4.1   Japanese girdle wrap – 'sarashi'

Most midwives are aware of the importance of the deep abdominal muscles such as the internal obliques in supporting the spine as well as the abdomen and baby, and will advise on exercises such as the cat and simple abdominal work to support these muscles. This is working with the energy of the Girdle Vessel.

Traditionally, the Japanese would wear a girdle wrap during the pregnancy. You have to remember that they would be wearing kimonos which fastened round the waist with a belt, obi. They have small, slim bodies and would have been doing physical work which would keep the abdominal muscles strong. I am not necessarily suggesting that all women wear some form of girdle in pregnancy, but it can be useful to consider whether they need support at particular times. Interestingly, a version of the girdle is worn by women suffering from symphysis pubis diastasis so they can continue to do some activities. In Japan SPD is hardly known. The other way to provide support is to work the Girdle Vessel and Conception Vessel meridians.

The traditional wrap or 'sarashi' would first be worn on a special day around the 16–19th week of pregnancy; this is known as 'dog day' because dogs are supposed to have easy births and the dog spirit can protect and take away bad fortune. The mother would either wrap it herself or get her husband or other family member to do so. She would look more pregnant and announce her pregnancy from this time on. Each night she would take it off and rewrap it in the morning (Fig. 4.2). She would keep doing this till about 1 month after the birth. It was said to help the mother feel fetal movement and to warm the baby in a cold winter, as well as helping the mother's posture and easing backache. The lines of wrapping support both the Conception Vessel and Girdle Vessel.

These days, modern Japanese women don't have the time to keep wrapping, but many of them do wear types of corset during their pregnancies.

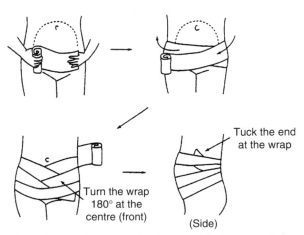

Figure 4.2   Girdle wrap (from Shusanki no rinshosyugi – Japanese Journal of Perinatal Care 106. Medicus Shuppan Publishing 2002, Japan, with permission).

Tuck the end at the wrap

Turn the wrap 180° at the centre (front)

(Side)

Heart–Uterus

This is closely linked with the energy of the Penetrating Vessel and is very much about Blood and emotional energy being settled or unsettled in the body. In the first trimester, the fetus may not make full use of Blood energy sent to it and this can be a cause of nausea and anxiety. As the fetus begins to grow more, it makes use of the Blood; nausea ceases and the mother becomes less anxious and more emotionally connected with her baby. Heart–Uterus is about the combination of earth and fire energy (see below).

Kidney–Uterus

The fetus draws on the Essence supplied to it via this meridian. This means that the mother may feel coldness in the Kidneys, suffer from lower backache and feel tired. It is closely linked with effects on Kidney energy and with all the extraordinary vessels as they share this internal pathway.

Kidney–Uterus is about the combination of earth and water energy (see below).

Effects on the 12 organs and meridians

Do turn back to the functions of the organs/meridians on pages 43–49 to get more of an idea of what they will affect both emotionally and physically in pregnancy.

Kidneys and Bladder – water

These are, in a sense, the most important organs/meridians as they are linked with Yin, Essence and body fluids. With so much Essence and Blood focused on nourishing the fetus, the mother may suffer from not having enough Yin energy. If the mother has good Kidney energy and strong Essence, then she can feel well; but if there have already been demands made on her Kidney energy before the pregnancy, then she is likely to find it hard and there may be problems with the growth and development of her baby. This is often the scenario for women who are constitutionally weak, older women in their late 30s to early 40s (as with age there is less Essence), drug abusers, those who are overtaxed physically, emotionally and sexually, or those who have suffered for a long time from chronic disease.

Women who have conceived through fertility treatments have undergone an overstimulation of their Kidney energy in order to conceive, and it is often the case that they experience a depletion of their Kidney energy during the pregnancy itself. If a woman has lots of children, especially close together, then Kidney energy (and also Uterus) can get depleted.

Excessive physical work may weaken Kidney Yang energy which will fail to transform and excrete fluids, so that they accumulate under the skin causing oedema. Moderate physical work is fine and may even minimize oedema. Overwork places a strain on Kidney energy, and these days many women are working excessively. This may lead to stress and other conditions to do with the flow of fluids such as urine (e.g. urinary tract infections, cystitis, blood flow). Hypotension and hypertension can both be linked with the Kidney. Weak Kidney energy can also affect the Lungs as they can fail to help Lung energy move down the body.

If the mother doesn't have enough Yin energy, then she can have too much Yang energy which tends to rise. Yang energy rising is often expressed through wood energy. The Kidneys are closely related to the Liver – water needs to nourish wood to allow it to grow and be flexible. If the Kidneys fail to nourish the Liver, then its energy can rise to the head. This is the energetic pattern behind the aggravation of migraine in some women. The ultimate collapse of Kidney energy in the mother is pre-eclampsia (or eclampsia) which is linked with blinding headaches and tightening pain in the abdomen – an expression of Liver energy.

The Bladder energy relates to the normal functioning of the uterus and autonomic nervous system, as well as to supporting the spine through the erectae spinae muscles. Weakness and backaches are often linked with low Bladder or Kidney energy.

If the mother can tune into the watery state of pregnancy and 'go with the flow', resting as she needs to and not pushing herself too hard, she can feel quite well. It is the tension set up by always being on the go and especially by being in stressful situations that draws upon adrenal energy, and this will cause tension in the Kidney and Bladder meridians.

Emotionally, water energy is linked to the mother's ancestral or family energy. It is a time when women often feel drawn to healing their relationships with family members, to connecting with and understanding their past, where they have come from and how the new baby is going to be part of this picture. In cultures where we don't have this sense of family connection, the mother can feel isolated and is more prone to stress, as well as even feelings of rejection towards her baby, feeling that it is a burden too great to bear on her own.

Spleen/Stomach – earth

Earth energy is a key energy of pregnancy – it is about both physical and emotional nourishment. Earth provides the soil for the seed, the baby, to grow. In traditional societies, the mother would draw support from her family. It would often be her mother or grandmother who would act as the midwife. The importance of this type of family support cannot be underestimated and is an expression of earth energy. The mother needs to be nourished emotionally, 'mothered', surrounding herself with people who will take care of her needs in practical ways, especially cooking her food. She needs to have good physical nourishment, so she can enjoy the roundness and fullness of pregnancy – earth energies. However, in our culture, there is pressure for a woman to appear not to be pregnant, to remain slim and slender rather than round and curvy, and many women worry about putting on too much extra weight. This creates tension and may cause the mother to feel disconnected from her real needs and frustrated with the pregnancy. If she does put on too much weight, especially by eating too much sugar, which affects the Spleen, she can feel very stuck and burdened down emotionally, as well as physically.

Extra demands are placed on the Spleen because of pregnancy being a Yin state, which means that there are more fluids in the body, including Blood. Since the Spleen generates and transforms the Blood energy, the increased demand for Blood after conception to nourish the fetus may result in the Spleen's function of promoting transportation and transformation declining. This can lead to problems of puffiness and oedema, especially in the legs, as well as digestive problems. Poorly functioning Spleen can be a cause of gestational diabetes or blood sugar problems. A faulty diet, especially eating greasy or dairy foods, worry, excessive thinking and fatigue all weaken the Spleen and aggravate these conditions.

As the baby grows, it tends to block the mother's energy in her groin, which prevents the Spleen meridian flowing in the legs, placing further demands on it. Conditions such as varicose veins in the legs, or vulval varicosities or haemorrhoids are related to the Spleen not being able to hold the blood in the blood vessels.

The changes in the size of the mother and the stretching of the flesh, especially along the midline of the body, mean that the Spleen has to work hard at its function of keeping organs in place. If it fails, then there may be prolapse of any abdominal organ. Heavy, dragging-down feelings in any muscle, but especially in the abdomen, often relate to the Spleen.

As the blood volume increases through the pregnancy, there are increased demands placed on the Spleen. The mother may become anaemic. In pregnancy, this cannot be said to be caused by a deficiency of Blood energy – there is more Blood energy as menses has ceased. This links with the Western viewpoint that while there is an increase in blood volume, and also an increase in the absolute number of red blood cells, there are fewer red blood cells relative to the larger increase in blood volume. This means there is a fall in haemoglobin concentration which is considered normal and signifying good expansion in blood volume not true anaemia. In some cases the haemoglobin levels may drop excessively and the mother may become anaemic. This is often resolved by improving the diet – that is to say by nourishing the Stomach and Spleen so they can make Blood.

Spleen weakness can mean that the energy of the Stomach, which needs to go down to help digestion and grounding, rises up. This aggravates the rising of the Penetrating Vessel energy in the first trimester which we discussed earlier.

If Stomach Ki fails to descend, stagnant food may accumulate in the stomach. Later in pregnancy, this may lead to problems with digestion such as heartburn.

Case study 4.2   Shiatsu in pregnancy by a midwife shiatsu practitioner

L is a midwife and also a shiatsu practitioner. She worked with client J, aged 37, who came for weekly sessions of shiatsu from 34 weeks. Here is a summary of the themes she was working with.

'J came for relaxation, and to focus on her own needs and the baby. I felt that an important part of the sessions was to connect with the Kidney/Uterus and the baby. I also treated the Conception Vessel and Governing Vessel in most sessions. J found the most enjoyable parts of the treatment were when I worked on the Conception Vessel over the Uterus and connected with the Kidney–Uterus. She was amazed by how relaxed and quiet the baby was during the treatments. As the baby was otherwise very busy, this in itself added to the relaxation she experienced.

At the second session, her Ki was concentrated in her lower body, with water presenting itself as overactive and the Spleen being more depleted. My impression was that depleted earth was unable to control the water. By the third session, wood presented itself as overactive with earth Kyo. Ki was concentrated in her upper body, with her whole body feeling very stiff and heavy. Her feelings of heaviness may also have been due to excess fluids (shown for example by a puffy face) and the Spleen not being able to fully transform fluids resulting in excess damp. I used more vigorous treatment to move the stuck wood but it also felt appropriate to spend time supporting her depleted Spleen energy.

Much of the shiatsu in the sessions was focused on tonifying depleted earth and Kidney energy. By tonifying earth energy in the sessions, J was able to focus more on herself and her own needs. My impression was that her busy family life had prevented her from focusing on the pregnancy and herself, thus depleting her energy. She felt that shiatsu helped to ease her stiffness and 'heaviness' thus helping her to feel more comfortable. By the final session, the cycle of energy had moved from wood into fire with J focusing on preparing for the birth of the baby. During this session J talked about where in her house she would like to give birth, what she would need for the birth and said that she had already started getting clothes ready for the new baby. Much of the work in this session was to tonify her depleted earth rather than disperse the fire.

J felt that shiatsu had helped her to feel well and energized during the latter part of the pregnancy, and that shiatsu had helped to balance her energy.'

Heart and Small Intestine – fire

Fire is the ruler of all emotions and linked with the Shen (Spirit). It is the Yang energy of pregnancy. If the mother feels happy with her pregnancy, she can focus on her positive bond and developing relationship with her baby, as well as her changing relationship with her partner. She needs to be able to express her feelings about what is going on – her joys and sadnesses, to feel emotionally supported, and then fire energy can flow.

Ideally, the mother should feel safe from anxiety in her pregnancy. Unfortunately, in modern culture, the incidence of violence against women increases in pregnancy, partly because the partner's Heart energy is affected by the changing relationship (Andrews & Brown 1988, Bohn 1990, Sweet 1997). This affects the mother's Heart energy and can lead to depression, either antenatally or postnatally. Severe shock can also weaken the constitution of the baby, as well as creating an emotional and physical predisposition to anxiety.

Physically, the Heart energy has to work harder in pregnancy because of the increased blood volume; this means that emotionally heart energy can be less stable and it rises easily in pregnancy. The mother may feel overly hot or ungrounded and unstable. Excessive consumption of hot, spicy foods can turn into fire and disturb the Mind (Shen). Sadness and overwork weaken Heart energy, as does not sleeping well. The main fire meridians are in the arms and are regulated by the upper burner.

Triple Heater and Heart Protector – supplemental fire

Emotionally, these are about how the mother can integrate the changes of the pregnancy. They are related to the overall flow of energy in the body through their connections with the fascial system, particularly the immune and lymphatic systems, and the regulation of body temperature. Flowing in the arms, they are often involved with carpal tunnel syndrome or oedema in the arms, along with the Lung.

The Triple Heater controls normal mucus secretion in the uterus, and dampness in the lower burner can be a cause of infertility. It is said that the energy of the three burners gets blocked by the growing baby in the womb (lower burner area) which then affects digestion as well as respiration and elimination functions (see page 53 for more information on this).

Liver and Gall Bladder – wood

Wood energy is about growth and new life, and needs physical activity to keep it flowing. In our culture, most women are not engaged in much physical activity and this tends to block wood energy which gathers in the neck, jaw, head and shoulders, causing emotional and physical tension. This is aggravated by sitting at a desk where the shoulders are often held stiffly. Rising wood energy may create heat and headaches. Blocked wood energy may cause feelings of frustration – unexpressed emotion. This often links in with the patterns of fire energy rising, and may create explosive emotional outbursts of frustration.

Wood energy likes to be in control and have an overview of the situation. The mother wants to know all the time what is happening with the baby and may feel that she is being taken over by someone else.

Liver stores the Blood and has a close relationship with the Penetrating Vessel – the Sea of Blood. In early pregnancy, when menstruation ceases, Blood and Ki tend to build up in the Liver and then the excess energy flows up the body. This aggravates the upward flow of the Penetrating Vessel, making the patterns of nausea more extreme, sometimes resulting in vomiting and even hyperemesis.

Progesterone and relaxin affect the ligaments/tendons which are ruled by the Liver; the instability of many of the major joints in the body can be said to be linked to Liver energy not supporting them. In the case of symphysis pubis diastasis, this may be linked to the Liver's relationship to the Girdle Vessel and also to excessive physical activity in the past which has caused the ligaments and tendons to become overstretched.

Lung and Large Intestine – metal

Emotionally, the Lungs relate to our sense of self and to how we perceive ourselves in the world. Our basic identity is often challenged in pregnancy and work with these meridians can help the mother to process these changes. The metal type can be emotionally detached – quite incisive and clear but often cold. Metal represents the movement toward Yin energy. Often these people find it hard or don't want to form close, emotional friendships, so they may lack support or be unable or unwilling to express their emotions. Since becoming a mother brings new emotions, they may find this time of life difficult to relate to – especially as it often brings with it a certain amount of letting go and lack of order, both of which the metal type finds hard to cope with.

The Lung has to work harder as respiration needs to expand in order to increase oxygenation and elimination and to take in more Ki. This means that the Lung energy tends to get quite stuck which affects the arms, sometimes resulting in carpal tunnel syndrome or oedema. Deep breathing, and shiatsu and exercise to open the chest will help Lung energy to flow better.

Physically, Lung types are often quite angular people and may find the roundness of pregnancy uncomfortable – they may be the kind of people who seem detached from their baby, or even not appear to be pregnant till quite late on.

The Large Intestine performs its role less effectively because of the compression from the growing baby and the effects of relaxin.

Energy patterns for the baby

The baby's energy is very much linked with the mother's, and this idea is expressed in the Eastern ideas of Tai Kyo – fetal education. There are theories about the development of the meridians in the baby and what is happening at each month. I will not go into these, as they don't easily relate to what we know about embryological development and need in-depth study (Matsumoto & Birch 1988). The most important energy shift is along the midline of the body – the development of the extraordinary vessels, which was discussed earlier (pages 35–36).

Main energy changes in labour

Birth is essentially a movement of energy from Yin, the state of pregnancy with the baby on the inside in water, to Yang, bringing the baby out into the world. The most Yin energy is water and the most Yang is fire. To move from Yin to Yang means to move into the season of spring, to the wood energy of growth and transformation. Wood is the movement of energy in the second stage of labour.

With the beginning of labour, there is a Yang, active impetus, caused by changes in the Governing Vessel. The first stage of labour is more Yin in relation to the second stage. The more Yin-type person will find the first stage of labour easier as Yin energy still predominates. As labour progresses to the second stage, she may find this more difficult. It is the opposite for the Yang-type person, who may well find the first stage of labour more difficult than the second stage.

Once the baby is born, it begins to form relationships with people other than its mother and this is more to do with fire energy, the most Yang energy. The mother also has to draw on her fire energy to relate to the baby in a different way, and on her metal energy to let go of the identity she had formed of her baby and relate to it as a separate person.

Main energy patterns for the mother in labour

As birth is a time of great change, which involves strong movements of the mother's Ki, Essence and Blood, the overall process is said to be regulated by the Governing and Conception Vessels. They regulate the hormonal changes and also send energy to the relevant meridians. As the Governing Vessel is related to the neocortex, its energy is about the movement to the more Yang energy of the second stage. The Conception Vessel relates to Yin energy and the old, instinctive aspects of the brain. If women are allowed to take instinctive positions in early labour, they are often curled in all fours or in fetal-type positions, with the Conception Vessel on the inside of their body, and the Yin energies protected by the Governing Vessel on the outside. As the mother progresses to the more Yang second stage, she may well begin to assume upright positions and engage the Yang energy of the Governing Vessel. This is the surge of catecholamines which happens in late first stage to cause the 'fetal ejection

reflex' (Newton 1987, Odent 1992). At this stage, many women can exhibit fear or anger – this indicates the emotions connected with the shift from water (fear) to wood (anger) energy which the mother is passing through.

Energy needs to move down to the perineum for the second stage, and this is connected with the lower pathways of the Governing Vessel and Conception Vessel. Governing Vessel energy needs to flow freely to allow the coccyx to move.

The Heart–Uterus needs to send Blood energy and the Kidney–Uterus needs to send Essence to the uterus. These energies can support a tired or ineffectively contracting uterus, as well as enable the baby to have these energies for its journey. They both help to settle the mother's and baby's emotions to aid them in processing the huge changes which are happening to them, and they help the mother stay connected with her baby. This focus is often particularly useful in the current climate of birth where so much emphasis is placed on coping with the pain of labour rather than supporting the baby in labour. Women often find this shift of focus helpful and they may even enjoy giving birth.

The Girdle Vessel affects changes in the pelvis – if it is too loose then the contractions may be ineffective, if it is too tight then the baby may get stuck. There can be a big difference in energy from front to back. Sometimes, with ineffective contractions, there can be too much energy in the lower back and not enough flowing round to the uterus. This may cause or be caused by the baby being in an unhelpful position. Sometimes the pattern can be the reverse and then the mother would feel excessive pain in her abdomen. The Girdle Vessel can help direct the energy of the abdomen, particularly the deep abdominal muscles, to assist with bearing down in the second stage.

The energy of water (Kidney and Bladder) – first stage

This is the energy of the first stage of labour. The latent phase is more to do with the still water quality but as labour gathers momentum, it is the expression of the more Yang aspects of water – the strong flowing river that gradually gathers momentum and power as labour progresses. The prostaglandins stimulate contractions and relate to water. Stress affects prostaglandin production (water element). If water doesn't flow, then the mother can feel like she is in a pool of stagnant water and this state is characterized by fear and trembling. It is known that fear is the main emotion that can block the first stage as it triggers the adrenal response and the release of catecholamines such as epinephrine and norepinephrine which relate to Kidney energy. These hormones shunt blood from the uterus and placenta, slow down contractions and decrease oxygen to the fetus. The mother needs to be in a stress-free

---

Case study 4.3   Working to support the water energy of first stage – a midwife trained in shiatsu skills, labour ward

'E was in labour, admitted at 41 weeks for induction because of post-dates. Her contractions were every 2 to 3 min and very strong. The doctors had been in the room to look at her cardiotacography as the midwife caring for her had been concerned about some decelerations of the fetal heart. However, these had settled and were judged to be a result of compression of her baby's head, hopefully a sign of progress.

The entrance of the doctors had created fear for E who had until then been managing the pain of the contractions very well. She had now become tense and her breathing pattern had altered. She said that she was afraid that her baby was going to die; that she could feel there was something wrong.

I spent some time reassuring E that her baby's heartbeat was fine. She had had some diamorphine and said that she felt 'out of control'. This was stated in a calm manner but with certainty.

I asked E if I could try working with some shiatsu points to help her feel calmer and she agreed.

I began by stroking along her Bladder meridian in a downward direction to promote a sense of courage and vitality, and along the Governing Vessel which influences our nervous and mental condition. E said that she was feeling more relaxed. I showed the midwife who was looking after E and E's husband how to work along these meridians.

I then applied gentle pressure to SP-6 (see Section 3). Pressure at this point can have the effect of calming the spirit. E now seemed much more relaxed. Her baby's heartbeat was good so I left her in the care of her midwife.

This case study shows how the involvement of the doctors, or possibly any potential problem, can have quite a profound effect on the coping mechanisms of a woman in labour, creating fear and apprehension. Fear, stress and altered breathing patterns, such as breath-holding, have been shown to subsequently affect the progress and outcomes of labour. Also the mother's memory of labour will be marred by this experience of fear.

---

environment to allow water to flow and maybe it is this instinctive connection with water energy that has led to the increase in popularity of water births – or at least the use of water for pain relief during the first stage of labour. Women who have an affinity with water energy will tend to find the first stage of labour easy, but may find it hard to shift to the more Yang energy of the second stage.

The energy of wood (Gall Bladder and Liver) – second stage

This is about an increase of Yang energy – the water energy moving to wood energy – which needs to move down to the perineum to enable the baby to be born. Wood energy is stimulated by the release of oxytocin produced by the posterior pituitary gland which relates to the Governing Vessel.

Strong wood energy is physically demanding and women who have been sedentary may find its power too strong. The tendency for wood energy is to get stuck in the shoulders, and often at transition it is noticeable how women can clench their jaws, hold their breath and feel quite angry – all of which are expressions of wood energy being stuck. A person whose wood energy is flowing well tends to like the feelings of second stage and at last of being able to be more active and more in control of what is going on. It is known that opening the eyes may help focus in the second stage (Simkin & Ancheta 2000) and the eyes relate to wood energy.

As wood types typically like to be in control, then they may find they don't like the unpredictability of labour and having a baby. They may find the first stage of labour difficult as it is about opening up and allowing energy to flow freely, like water. Women often say they like to feel in control of labour – but what they really mean is that they are able to do what they want and can make the decisions that need to be made. Wood can be over-controlling – an expression of this would be a woman who wanted to know how long labour was going to last, how many more contractions she was going to have, when her baby was going to be born, rather than simply staying with the energy of each contraction.

Case study 4.4   Moving from water to wood – a midwife trained in shiatsu skills, labour ward

'I was asked by the midwife caring for this lady to come in to help with pain relief and relaxation. S was gravida 2, 41 weeks. S was very distressed, in advanced labour and appeared to me to be approaching the transitional stage. She had been 7 cm dilated at the last vaginal examination. S was lying on her left side.

During the contractions her shoulders were around her ears and she was extremely tense. She was using nitrous oxide.

At this stage of labour, it is very difficult to introduce yourself and to expect the woman to trust you; however S was desperate for support. Her husband was holding her hand.

I rested my hands on her shoulders for a little while and as I felt them start to rise with the contraction, began to encourage her to drop them a little. This had no effect the first time. Then I explained to S what she could do to help herself, and that I would help her and we would try again with the next contraction. I held my hands lightly on her shoulders and encouraged her to keep them low and relaxed throughout the contraction (*stuck wood energy beginning to release*). This was more successful. After a few contractions, she said that this was helping her. Would I stay?

She appeared to be more in control. While holding her shoulders, my intention was in a downward direction and the aim was to relax her shoulders, neck and jaw. My hands were covering GB-21 (wood point – see Section 3) but I was not directly pressing these points.

Between some of the contractions, I held my hands over her lower abdomen and lower back, focusing on S's breath and the baby. This appeared to have a comforting effect. I did not use sacral pressure, as S's pain was more concentrated at the front, above the symphysis pubis. I also used finger pressure on GV-20 (Governing Vessel point, directing Yang energy down, see Section 3) with downward focused intention to help relax the neck and shoulders and hopefully the vagina.

Very soon she had urges to push.

Her baby's head was slow to deliver. This can sometimes indicate a possible shouder dystocia and with S's history we were prepared for this possibility. There was some difficulty with her baby's shoulders, but with S in the McRoberts position they were born with the next contractions. A lovely girl, Apgar 8 and weighing 4500 kg. S was reluctant to part with her placenta (she had been given syntometrine). 20 min had passed. This was not very long. However, there was no sign of separation, which would be expected at this point. A urinary catheter was passed to empty her bladder, routine in this circumstance. Still no sign of separation.

Her baby was on her chest, skin to skin, but not ready to suckle.

The next step would then be a vaginal examination to feel for the placenta at the os, so I asked if I could try some shiatsu.

I applied pressure to GB-21, both shoulders, with S's permission.

The midwife who was caring for S mentioned that she could see the cord wiggle and began controlled cord traction (CCT) again. The placenta was still firmly attached; I applied more pressure to GB-21 as the midwife applied CCT. The placenta and membranes were then delivered, complete.

I feel that shiatsu was very helpful for S, even though it was given so late in her labour. I believe that her memory of the birth will be more positive.

She was able to help herself, which I think is very important.

My colleague's responses were positive throughout. She had asked me to come into the room to help. She appeared impressed with the effect of GB-21. There was a student midwife present who was very interested in the shiatsu and the relaxation aspects of the care. I could have shown her husband some points to use and some simple techniques. He was very supportive and would have felt even more involved'.

The energy of fire (Heart/Small Intestine/Triple Heater and Heart Protector) – third and 'fourth' stages

Third stage is very similar energy to second stage but less intense. It is still about the downward movement of the wood energy to deliver the placenta. If this doesn't happen, then the placenta may be retained. You will have read about this in case study 4.4. However, there is already a shift of movement from wood to fire which happened with the birth of the baby, and the mother's and baby's energy is more expansive. This is the energy of the fourth stage – the beginning of the bonding process between the mother and her baby.

Fire energy in labour is about providing emotional support to women in labour and allowing them to be able to express their feelings, especially if they get stuck. Feelings of connection with the baby and focus on the baby can be very useful for them – which can involve working with the Heart–Uterus meridian.

The energy of metal – Lung and Large Intestine

These are important as they relate to letting go – which is what the mother is doing with her baby. It is the first stage in the separation process which will happen with mother and baby, until

---

Case study 4.5   Earth energy – mother energy, the energy of the home and touch. A natural birth clinic in Japan – Yae, a Japanese shiatsu practitioner

I studied acupuncture, moxa and massage for 3 years at Toyo Shinkyu Senmon Gakko in Shinjuku, from which I graduated in 1994. But the massage I learnt in school was too 'general' for me, so I went to learn Masunaga Shiatsu (Zen shiatsu) at Iokai in Tokyo in 1995. I fell in love with the power of Zen shiatsu, and so I have since stopped practising acupuncture in my treatment.

From my happy experience of my first natural birth at the Huang Midwife Clinic, and being aware of the amazingly warm atmosphere that Sugiyama-sensei (and her assistant midwives) was creating, I wanted to be involved in this wonderful maternity world through my work. This kind of clinic is very rare in Japan now. I have heard of the names of a few other clinics which use the natural methods like Huang, but I still think Huang is a very special place even among them. Something like 95% of Japanese women choose birth at ordinary (Western-type) hospitals, which sounds terrible to me. Those mothers, who chose Huang, mostly had a strong belief in natural living and natural/oriental treatments, which made my work very easy and enjoyable.

The clinic is a small place – Sugiyama's house – and a small number of dedicated young midwives work for a small salary. They are responsible for nearly everything happening in the clinic from day to night – cooking meals, cleaning the house, washing and hanging, making sure that someone is always there to be ready for the mothers' needs. You sleep on a futon (there are no beds), sometimes side by side with other mothers if it is a busy period. Even the next room is divided only by a Japanese paper sliding door so there is not much privacy. And everybody – sensei, midwives, and mothers – eats together in the dining/living room. So it is indeed like a one big family, so safe, so warm. While you stay there for 4 days, sleeping together and eating together, sharing one's most exciting experience of life, you'll make a friend for life.

That's why most mothers come back to the clinic for the next baby. Once you have experienced the incredible warm energy at the clinic, you would not think of any other place. Sugiyama-sensei, aged about 55, is just a humble, gentle lady, but she attracts everybody. I do not know where her power comes from.

Kindly, Sugiyama-sensei gave me a chance to work in the clinic by running a semi-weekly 'moxa class' for pregnant women; she also introduced me to clients (pre- and postnatal) who were interested in receiving my shiatsu treatment. Nearly all the mothers who were going to have a baby at the clinic were encouraged to attend the moxa class after their fifth month of pregnancy and received instructions on the acupoints (mainly 'san-in-kou' SP-6) and how to do moxa by themselves.

My prenatal clients came to me for back pain, leg pain, breech baby, constipation, tiredness, piles, morning sickness, stiff shoulders, sleeping disorder, and also merely for comfort and security (believing shiatsu ensures them an easy labour). The postnatal clients came to me for abdomen pain after labour, numbed legs, back pain, piles, lacking breast milk, tiredness, constipation, stiff shoulders and stiff arms, etc. But I did not do baby massage, nor breast massage; and I've never done shiatsu in the labour room either.

I applied a whole-body Zen shiatsu course to the client first. Then, even though Zen shiatsu does not talk about particular acupoints, I often prefer to use 'moxa' as well to the particular acupoints that are effective for particular symptoms (e.g. SP-6 for nearly every symptom, 'shi-in' (BL-67) in the Bladder meridian for breech baby, and 'hyaku-e' (GV-20) in the governing meridian for piles) (see Section 3 for more information on these points).

I have seen a lot of cases where the client's body has changed to a more relaxed, flexible one by giving shiatsu, so I am sure shiatsu is good for maternity care. Most of all, I feel that shiatsu is particularly important for people who need more comfort and support, like pregnant women, because the whole practice itself includes 'touching' people for such a long time, and 'giving' out your warm Ki energy. Through this kind of communication between clients and myself, I feel that I support them mentally as well, just like their midwives.

In this clinic, midwives use some kind of very basic massage techniques, e.g. rubbing the lower back of a mother experiencing contractions with some herb oils, and also giving moxa/or finger pressure on SP-6 to induce stronger contractions, and of course giving breast massage to postnatal mothers. They use lots of other kinds of natural resources which have traditionally been used in Japan, as well as wonderful home-made low-calorie meals made with traditional Japanese ingredients, cabbage/or mountain-yam pack for painful breasts with excessive milk, home-made honey–garlic paste drink for postnatal constipation.

Note: Moxa is a Japanese herb that is burnt near points to generate heat.

---

the baby as an adult leaves the mother and forges their own identity. Women may feel grief as well as joy in this process, and this grief can block labour as the mother on some level does not feel ready to let go of her baby.

Breath is important because of its connection with Lung and because it provides the air Ki necessary to support the process of labour which requires a lot of Ki.

The energy of earth – Stomach and Spleen

This provides the centre of the whole process and governs the energy of the strong muscular contractions. If earth energy is not flowing, women may feel emotionally stuck and find it difficult to get the impetus to go into labour. Once in labour, they should progress easily if in a supportive environment and are allowed to eat as they need to. They may need to sing and make sounds.

Moving women from one environment to another, as in the transfer from home to hospital, can unsettle the earth energy and may be why contractions stop. Unsettled earth energy may then affect all the other elements, especially water.

Baby's energy in labour

Introduction

The process of birth for the baby is about moving from the Yin water environment of the womb to the earth outside, and from being dependent on the mother's Ki, Blood and Essence for nourishment to making the transition to producing its own energies. The circuit of the extraordinary vessels is important in regulating this process of change. In the fetal position, the Governing Vessel is around the Conception and Penetrating Vessels. During labour, it is stimulated through compression and then undergoes changes at birth as the baby's spine is extended and the head and shoulders rotate.

Kidney – water

The baby responds to labour contractions by showing a rise in catecholamine (dopamine, epinephrine and norephinephrine) output from the adrenal medulla and from extramedullary cells. Umbilical arterial concentrations of these catecholamines are four times higher in vaginally delivered babies than those delivered by Caesarean (Sweet 1997). They provide a variety of cardiorespiratory and metabolic adaptations during and after labour, and relate to Kidney and extraordinary vessel energy. Water energy is about change and adaptation. It is particularly about the ability we have in our lives to be able to cope with stressful situations. There is some evidence that babies born by Caesarean find it more difficult to go through stress and spend their lives either trying to avoid it or create it (Chamberlain 1988, Emerson, unpublished work, 1996).

Lung – metal

During the last couple of days before labour begins, fetal breathing activity is reduced and lung liquid is produced at a gradually decreasing rate. This is linked with the increase in catecholamines. There is a difference in lung function between babies born vaginally and those born by Caesarean – higher levels of surfactant and more rapid elimination of lung liquid occurs in response to the stimulatory effects of labour (Irestedt et al 1982, Mortola et al 1982, Oliver 1981, Sweet 1997). This is why Caesarean babies are often quite mucousy.

Problems during birth that affect fetal oxygenation or delay the onset of normal respiration, such as prolonged labour, malposition of the fetus, excessively narrow pelvic outlet, placental insufficiency and problems with the umbilical cord, can cause Ki to become trapped in the Lungs. This may lead to problems with Lung Ki in infancy and later life such as a wide variety of respiratory and allergic disorders, as well as identity issues. The old practice of slapping the baby on the back at birth would further complicate this by sending the Ki trapped in the Lungs to the Heart. The effect on the Heart is to cause nervousness, irritability, restless sleep and low energy in the child and indeed these Heart patterns may continue in later life.

A study by Salk et al (1985) suggested a link between respiratory distress for more than 1 h at birth and the increased incidence of adolescent suicide. This fits in with the Chinese view of Heart and Lung Ki being affected at birth and setting up long-term patterns of imbalance in the organs and meridians.

Heart – fire

Birth is about the baby meeting the outside world and forming relationships, both a different relationship with the mother and new relationships with others. This relates to the Heart and supplemental fire – Heart Protector and Triple Heater. Until the baby is born, it is the mother who protects the baby's heart energy – in a sense, the mother is the baby's Heart Protector and Triple Heater. Problems at birth which affect the cardiovascular system will affect both the Heart and Lungs, as seen above. If the Heart is affected, then, as an adult, the person may have a tendency to feel tired, emotionally labile, unstable, hot tempered or even feel inexplicably anxious and nervous.

Understanding the changes in the early postnatal period

Main energy changes for the mother

Some schools of thought say that as the antenatal period is 9 months, it also takes 9 months postnatally for the body to recover. In many traditional cultures, the period of full recovery was much longer and women were advised to wait 5–7 years to have another child (Goldsmith 1984). This fits in with the idea of Essence flowing in 7-year cycles – it needs time to replenish its quality.

In traditional Japan there was an initial rest period of 21 days (toko age 21 nichi) and many women still observe this. If the mother had given birth in the midwife's house, she would be looked after by her and given special foods, shiatsu would be given to the mother and the baby as needed. The midwife would often massage the mother's breast or show her how to massage them, to help with milk flow and prevent mastitis. There used to be many special Japanese masseurs who specialized in breast massage before and after birth. These days there are not so many but they still exist. They tend to work directly on the breasts with white sesame oil. This may sound horrible, but our culture tends to ignore the breasts when doing massage and shiatsu. In my courses, I often encourage practitioners to experiment with different kinds of touch and massage to the breast in a non-sexual way, and to a level of comfort that is appropriate in the situation. Usually, people are surprised how relaxing it can be. For a mother who has engorged breasts, appropriate massage and shiatsu can feel wonderful. This will be described in Section 3. Women can choose to have the shiatsu done directly on the skin or may feel more comfortable with work done through the clothes. If they prefer to do it themselves, then they can be shown the techniques.

Table 4.1 The decline of breastfeeding in Japan (Maternal and Child Health Statistics of Japan 2001)

Statistics for breastfeeding	1–2 months	2–3 months	3–4 months
In 1960	70.5%	62.1%	56.4%
In 2000	44.8%	42.3%	39.4%

Case study 4.6   Breast massage in Japan

Andrea is an Austrian shiatsu practitioner who had her first baby in Japan in 1990. She chose to engage an elderly traditional midwife and gave birth in the midwife's house.

'Samba san massaged me in the next 2 days (after the birth). She put warm and wet towels on my breasts and started directly massaging my breasts one after the other, trying to make the milk flow and enhance milk production. She also cooked for me – she gave me fish soup, fish, rice and vegetables – she told me these are things that make the milk flow well'.

In traditional Japan, women would tend to breastfeed for 1–2 years, taking the baby with them to the field. Now, like most modern industrialized cultures, more women in the cities are beginning to work outside the home after only a few weeks with the baby, and breastfeeding rates are declining. Traditionally women would continue to wear the girdle wrap (see p. 55) for at least 1 month postnatally.

The force required for delivery draws upon the woman's Ki – especially wood. The loss of blood during birth drains Blood and Yin. The expulsion of the placenta uses original Ki. All these mean that a deficiency of Ki, Blood and Yin are the overriding conditions of women after childbirth. The Conception and Penetrating Vessels are depleted; the blood vessels and channels are empty and prone to invasions by external factors such as cold, heat, infection. Even if the mother had an easy birth and feels well immediately afterwards, it is still important for her to make sure that she looks after herself in the first few weeks to allow her energies to replenish themselves. Unfortunately, it is common these days for women to feel pressurized to 'get back to normal'. If they don't get enough rest early on, they are drawing on their deeper reserves of energy, especially their Essence. Longer term, they are more likely to suffer from exhaustion.

Depletion of Ki

Sweating, fever and exhaustion are signs of depleted Ki. There will be persistent lochial discharge which is red, profuse, dilute, with no smell.

In shiatsu, we would see which meridians and areas of the body were most depleted and work with those. The most depleted area is usually the hara, the abdomen, the result of the sudden change of no longer containing the baby and the laxity of the abdominal muscles. All the meridians which pass through the abdomen, especially the Conception Vessel and Penetrating Vessel, will be depleted in energy, as well as the lower back (Kidney and Governing Vessel) and the Girdle Vessel. This is why women wore the sarashi (girdle) to give support and bring more energy to this area.

For women who have had a Caesarean, the hara is cut through energetically and energy flows must be encouraged. It is important for the mother to do some gentle exercise to prevent stagnation of Ki, but not to do excessive exercise which would deplete her energy still further.

Depletion of Blood energy

There is said to be a loss of Blood energy with the discharge of the placenta and the resulting changes in the uterine lining. As the Penetrating Vessel is the sea of Blood energy, this channel will be depleted. Signs of deep depletion are heavy bleeding, excessive discharge of lochia and nausea. In this case, work needs to be done to replenish the Blood energy. Blood energy can get stuck in the uterus and in this case the lochial discharge is dark, purplish and with clots. In this case, work would need to be done to move the Blood energy, for example by gentle stretches and working away from the uterus. There can also be heat in the Blood energy which usually means heavier bleeding and the lochial discharge will be bright red or dark red, often with a foul smell. In this case, it is important not to use warming techniques, such as applying hot towels or the Chinese herb moxa, as these will aggravate the condition.

As Heart governs Blood energy, it is said that with the loss of Blood energy, the physical basis of the Heart, the Heart becomes restless as it has no anchor. Restless Heart energy rises, often to the head, and affects the Shen, the spirit, which it rules. This is the Chinese explanation of postnatal depression. The other main meridians connected with the Blood energy will also be affected – Spleen and Liver. It is important that the mother finds a balance between gentle exercise and rest to both move and restore Liver Blood energy.

It is considered that breast milk is a transformation of Blood energy, so if the mother's Blood energy is low, then the mother may not be able to produce enough milk.

Depletion of Yin

The loss of fluids may lead to there being insufficient Yin in the body, which means that the body can become too hot. If the mother is very hot, it is then important to avoid excessive exposure to heat, as sweating is weakening after birth. Exposure to cold is not recommended either as the Chinese considered it to be one of the main causes of postpartum problems.

Meridian patterns postnatally

Extraordinary Vessel energy

Penetrating vessel energy is the most important energy postnatally as it controls the breasts as well as the Blood energy. Its pathway fans out over the breasts and chest on its way to the throat and eyes – the breast connecting channels. These control the major arteries that feed the breast i.e. the axillary artery supplying the outer half and the internal mammary arteries supplying the inner half of the breast. Breast milk is seen as a transformation of Blood energy, so if the Penetrating Vessel is empty, the Sea of Blood energy is depleted and there may not be enough milk. If the Ki of the Penetrating Vessel is not flowing, then the breast connecting channels will be blocked and the milk may not flow even though it is abundant.

The Conception Vessel and Governing Vessel continue to be important in regulating the hormonal changes of the postnatal period. They are also linked with the changing energy of the abdomen and back. They are especially important as they allow energy to flow to the perineum and will help with perineal repair and the pelvic floor muscles. As Yin energy tends to be depleted, the Conception Vessel needs to be supported to nourish it, especially as the mother's energies are nourishing her baby. The Conception Vessel also promotes the movement of body fluids which include milk.

Yang energy also needs to flow postnatally. The milk ejection reflex linked with oxytocin is the same energetic circuit described in the second stage of labour – and is linked with the Governing Vessel and Gall Bladder energy.

The Girdle Vessel continues to play its role in supporting the pelvis and is often put out of balance by the mother holding the baby on one hip only. The Heart–Uterus and Kidney–Uterus support the changes in the Uterus.

Kidney and Bladder

As we have seen, Essence, stored in the Kidneys, has supported the whole process of pregnancy and birth and it takes 7 years for this energy to be replenished. It is important for the mother not to be in stressful situations, especially working long hours outside the home for some time, otherwise she will draw still further on her Essence. This needn't necessarily be the full cycle of 7 years, but for a few years, she will need to be careful of her energy. This includes ideally spacing children so Kidney energy has a chance to renew itself.

Stomach and Spleen

The Stomach influences breastfeeding as its pathway passes through the breast. Breast milk is a transformation of menstrual Blood energy which is supplemented by postnatal Ki extracted from food by the Stomach.

If the mother is not producing enough breast milk, it can be because of a depletion of her Blood energy. The Stomach and Spleen work with the Penetrating Vessel to help build up quality reserves of milk

Heart and Small Intestine, Triple Heater and Heart Protector

In Chinese terms, depression is related to the exertion and loss of Blood energy at birth. Since the Heart houses the Mind and governs Blood energy, Heart–Blood energy becomes deficient, the Mind has no residence and it becomes depressed and anxious. This causes a state of depression, mild anxiety, insomnia and fatigue. The mother feels unable to cope, she is tearful, she loses libido and may feel angry. In time, Blood energy deficiency may lead to Yin deficiency. In many women there is a mild version of this pattern. The more extreme puerperal psychosis would be seen as stagnant Blood energy harassing the Mind.

Heart energy is linked with the Heart Protector which then has more work to do. The Triple Heater helps the mother adapt to her changing role, new rhythms and different ways of relating to people.

Liver and Gall Bladder

For wood energy to flow, there must be some movement of the body. However, excessive exercise can draw too much on wood energy and so there is a need for gentle exercise combined with rest. Western views of postnatal exercise have varied over the years, but the Eastern view is based on this energetic understanding. Emotional problems such as worry or anger can affect Liver energy. Liver influences the breasts and controls the nipple, so it can obstruct the flow of milk. Posturally, Liver and Gall Bladder energy in the shoulders and the side of the neck tends to become quite tight – from the demands of holding and feeding a baby as well as sleeping awkwardly in bed at night. If Liver energy is not flowing it can cause constipation, as it fails to moisten the faeces.

Lung and Large Intestine

Blood deficiency and dryness affects the Large Intestine causing constipation, a common postnatal complaint, often leading to haemorrhoids. Sometimes this is caused by Lung Ki failing to descend to the Large Intestine to help it in its functions. If the mother postnatally does not breathe deeply and relax, then this will affect Lung functions. Often her posture will affect Lung energy – bent over the baby, feeding.

Emotionally, metal energy is about the process of defining oneself in the world and letting go. A woman's sense of self is challenged in this postnatal period. Metal represents money and our sense of worth – a woman's capacity to earn money is usually affected while having time off to look after the baby.

Main energy changes for the baby

At birth, the baby's Lung and Spleen need to start functioning so that they can produce their own Ki from food and air. The postnatal period for the baby is characterized by an even faster growth and development than occurred in the womb and an engagement with the earth. This is Yang energy. Yang energy is predominant until maturity and the peak activity of the body, which the Chinese consider to be around the age of 28. After this age, there is a movement towards old age and eventually death – Yang energy declines and Yin energy rises. Dying is the most Yin aspect of life and is about going back to the hidden realm and the universal energy.

During the first 6 months of a baby's life, its nervous system is affected by feeding patterns, quality and quantity of human contact, food, loud noise, and what the Chinese call 'pernicious influences' like wind, cold, wet, heat, dryness. Stresses are caused by the premature acceleration of a child's development, especially attempts to make the child stand and walk too early. Parents need to be encouraged to support and extend the baby's natural movements, rather than impose movement on them like in baby bouncers and walkers. Crawling in particular is a vital stage, as it makes links between the left and right sides of the brain.

Box 4.2

In Japan, like in most traditional cultures, the mother would go back to work in the fields quite soon after her baby was born, but carry the baby around with her. She wouldn't tend to undress the baby and massage her with oils because in winter it gets very cold. She would, however, often rub or hold points through the clothes. If the baby was upset she would rub her legs, or hold points.

Case study 4.7   Baby massage and shiatsu – Karen, midwife trained in shiatsu skills and massage

At the birth unit, we prepare parents for the adventure of parenthood through support groups, practical sessions and baby massage.

Baby massage is introduced after birth and the parents are shown simple strokes to do on their babies. Through gentle strokes and touch, the massage helps develop and relax the nervous system, which is a lovely way to relieve discomfort after birth, particularly after a long labour.

The ongoing baby massage classes I run with a colleague provide step-by-step massage strokes: gentle exercises to encourage coordination, and relaxation techniques that benefit both mum and baby.

Once a month we organize a session for fathers to come along and massage their babies and meet other dads. One father said 'It's a long time since I spoke your language but I am listening to you'.

We teach baby massage by demonstrating the strokes and encourage the parents to find their own special way to massage their baby. Eye contact and non-verbal cues are discussed.

In the baby massage sessions we also introduce simple shiatsu techniques such as holding the cranium and the coccyx to work the Conception and Governing Vessel to help accommodate the changes in the spine as the baby develops. It is also effective after birth when there has been compression on the head and neck, particularly in occipital posterior positions in labour.

Working on the feet can be very grounding for a baby, and we encourage the mothers to work between the toes to help move the energy and observe stress cues such as splaying of the toes.

When doing arm exercises, they gently cross the baby's arms across the chest, always watching how their baby responds. We demonstrate to the mother to hold both hands lightly over the baby's arms and chest, and rock back and forth; this is good for balancing the Governing Vessel.

For the parents, exercises are good to help them relax and release their tension from their bodies before working with their babies. Sometimes they go back to back with gentle rocking and stretching, or massage each other's shoulders or backs. This allows them time, which is so important with all the demands of being parents.

Extraordinary vessels – Conception Vessel and Governing Vessel

Passing through the spine and the front of the body, this circuit is very much affected by the process of birth and the movement from Yin to Yang. The uncurling from the fetal position and the development of the spine from the neck down, all reflect changes in the flow of this energy – this basic energy supporting all other meridian energies. The development of the digestive system is closely connected with the Conception Vessel.

Trauma at birth usually affects this midline, especially the Governing Vessel. In Caesareans, the spine is lifted out rather than compressed. Babies who are born by Caesarean miss out on the process of contraction and find it difficult to expel fluids, often suffering from congestive problems. Shiatsu work, introducing them to some gentle pressures, will help to get their energy flowing. Babies who are born by forceps/ventouse have excessive pressure placed on the skull and spine. This is not all that difficult to work with and it is better to support a baby to process the trauma as soon as possible, rather than allow it to be held as distorted energy flow for the rest of their life.

Lung

As the baby takes in its first breath, it begins to make its own Ki from the air and change the energy of the Lung. This links in with the emotional patterns of the baby having to relate to an external environment – beginning the establishment of its own identity as a person. Many babies, especially those born by Caesarean, suffer from slight snuffles and chesty conditions in this process of adaptation, and they are more susceptible to infections.

Stomach and Spleen

Sometime after taking in the first breath, the baby has to learn to take food in through the mouth rather than the umbilical cord. This is the taking in of food Ki through the Stomach. Birth weight doubles in the first 4 months and triples by 1 year. During the first year, the digestive system is working to maximum capacity to support this gain in weight and it is the Spleen that is responsible for digestion and absorption of food. Many muscles grow and develop and it is the Spleen that is responsible for this. The movement towards food strengthens the pathways of the Stomach and Spleen, the main pathways of the front of the body passing through the mouth.

Heart and Small Intestine, Triple Heater and Heart Protector

The baby has to begin to make relationships with people other than the mother. This draws on their fire energy. The Heart Protector and Triple Heater don't start functioning until birth, when the baby needs its own protection and heating. It takes time for these functions to establish themselves and so this is why, in the first few weeks, the baby is not able to regulate its own heating very well. The practices of wrapping and swaddling babies indicate the need to support this protective function of the Triple Heater and Heart Protector, which can also be achieved by keeping the baby close to the mother, who provided these functions while the baby was in the womb.

The practices of separating the baby from the mother and placing them in a nursery puts strain on these meridians and can set up an energetic pattern which can continue into adulthood of either having to overprotect themselves or disconnect from their painful emotions.

Bladder and Kidney

The spine muscle tone develops from the top down. At birth, there is no curvature of the spine – it forms one continuous curve. First, the cervical curvature develops, then later the lumbar curvature. This brings energy into these parts of the Governing Vessel and Bladder meridians. The spine is often affected by the birth process, especially Caesarean and forceps deliveries as we saw earlier.

Liver

In the early days, the Liver has to adapt to conjugate bilirubin. It is helpful to work with the Liver for jaundiced babies. As the baby is growing so much, and as they begin to be involved in physical activity, the Liver and Gall Bladder become very much involved.

Summary

We have now discussed the theory behind the different phases of pregnancy, birth and the postnatal period. In the next chapter we will explore how to put this into practice.

Reflect on the following:

Think of a woman you have worked with recently, where you were not sure what you could offer. Think of how you might apply some of your theory to identify what types of energy she needed supporting.

Do this for a woman in each of the phases of pregnancy, birth and in the early postnatal period.

REFERENCES

Andrews B, Brown G W 1988 Marital violence in the community. British Journal of Psychiatry 153:305–312

Bohn D K 1990 Domestic violence and pregnancy implications for practice. Journal of Nurse-Midwifery 35(2):86–98

Chamberlain D 1988 Babies remember bith and other extraordinary scientific discoveries about the mind and personality of your newborn. Jeremey Tarcher, USA

Goldsmith J 1984 Childbirth wisdom. Congden and Weed, New York

Irestedt L, Lagercrantz H, Hjemdahl P et al 1982 Fetal and maternal plasma catecholamine levels at elective caesarean section under general or epidural anaesthesia versus vaginal delivery. American Journal of Obstetrics and Gynecology 142(8):1004–1010

Maternal and Child Health Statistics of Japan 2001 Feeding of infant by age 1960–2000. Maternal and Child Health Division, Equal Employment, Child and Families Bureau, Ministry of Health, Labour and Welfare, Japan, p 126

Matsumoto K, Birch S 1988 Hara diagnosis, reflections on the sea. Paradigm Publications, Brookline, Massachusets, USA

Mortola J P, Fisher J T, Smith J B et al 1982 Onset of respiration in infants delivered by Caesarean section. Journal of Applied Physiology 52(3):716–724

Newton N 1987 The fetal ejection reflex revisited. Birth 14(2):106–108

Odent M 1992 The nature of birth and breastfeeding. Bergin & Garvey, Wesport, CT, USA

Oliver R E 1981 Of labour and the lungs. Archives of Diseases in Childhood 56:659–662

Salk L, Lipsitt L, Sterner W et al 1985 Relationship of maternal and perinatal conditions to eventual adolescent suicide. The Lancet 1(8429):624–627

Simkin P, Ancheta R 2000 The labour progress handbook. Blackwell Science, Oxford, p 88

Sweet B 1997 Mayes midwifery. Bailliere Tindall, London, p 351

Hands-on shiatsu – practical applications

'In order to understand meridians and tsubos, we must first feel inner life. Life itself is the cure of the disease. Also the trust that we can cure disease by life is most essential.' (Shitzuko Masunaga)

As we have seen from the previous section, shiatsu is about balancing different types of energy in the body, especially Yin and Yang. In this section, I look at the practical ways in which we can do this. Where possible, I draw out the links between shiatsu and what midwives may already do in their practice.

Chapter 5 will help you to identify the similarities and differences between shiatsu and other forms of bodywork. You will find that by learning these basic principles of touch, even without learning any specific meridians or points, you will be able to make any kind of bodywork more effective. Even if you have not understood all of the theory, you will notice a difference both in the way that you feel as you work with mothers and also in the quality of the work that you are doing. The simple techniques in this section can be easily taught in antenatal classes.

Chapters 6 and 7 build on from these basic principles to look at specific work suitable for pregnancy, labour and the postnatal period. They include some very simple techniques as well as more complicated ones. Remember that if you want to use the more complex techniques, or anything that is different from what you are instinctively doing, you will need to attend a course to make sure that what you are doing is correct.

5

Basic principles of shiatsu applications

Introduction

The hands-on skills of shiatsu are essentially instinctive and have developed over thousands of years. It is only a recent development of the last century for people to undergo formal training. Touch was an important part of how people related to each other day to day, as well being used in healing. I believe that many of the principles of shiatsu were probably in use in the West as well as the East, but with the much earlier industrializations in Europe, coupled with the witch hunts of the Middle Ages, these healing traditions were stamped out. What we are seeing in the 21st century, with the increase in popularity of Eastern ways of healing, is a re-integration into our culture of skills and knowledge which we probably had at one time but which have been lost. There will be aspects of shiatsu that midwives recognize as they are already using them as part of intuitive midwifery care. The aim of this section is to help you understand them better as well as to develop your skills.

I first want to look at some of the basic principles of shiatsu. This section will help you to identify the similarities and differences between shiatsu and other forms of bodywork. You will find that by learning these basic principles of touch, even without learning any specific meridians or points, you will be able to make any kind of bodywork more effective. Even if you have not understood all of the theory, you will notice a difference both in the way that you feel as you work with mothers and also in the quality of the work that you are doing. The simple techniques in this section can be easily taught in antenatal classes.

Shiatsu is not just about hands-on work. Shiatsu is about balancing the flow of energies in the body – mostly Ki and Essence. Ki, as you may remember from Chapter 3, comes from air and food. Air Ki is both about breathing and how we move oxygen around our body. Breath-work and exercise are therefore important aspects of shiatsu – both for the person receiving, as well as the person doing, the shiatsu so that their energy is balanced. As Ki is linked with the mind and emotions, visualization style techniques to connect with particular elements form part of shiatsu. Although food is also important, I am not going to discuss the role of diet as part of this book, as I feel it is too complex to cover this here, and there are many good books available on applying these principles (Pitchford 1993).

Box 5.1 Basic principles

- Be relaxed while doing shiatsu.
- Centre your attention on your hara (abdomen) and work from here.
- Work with penetrating perpendicular pressure not physical pressure.
- Work to balance Kyo and Jitsu – empty and full patterns.
- Use your two hands – mother hand, working hand principle.
- Work with continuity and flow.

I will now describe what these principles mean, as well as giving some exercises you can do, some on your own, but many with a partner. As 'hands-on' shiatsu is about contact with someone else, to experience what it is about, you need to work with someone else. Your partner could be a colleague, another midwife or a family member or friend. If you don't have any one to practise with, try to apply the principles as much as you can to your own body. You can do shiatsu on yourself, as I describe in Section 4.

Be relaxed

One of the most important principles is that there is an inter-relationship between the giver and the receiver: you the midwife and the mother. The way you feel when you are giving shiatsu will be transmitted to the mother. If you are feeling tense and uncomfortable, the work you do will be experienced by her as tense and uncomfortable. If you are holding your breath, she will hold her breath. If your energy is not flowing, her energy will not flow so well.

This may seem challenging to start with, but it is not that difficult to learn to use your body effectively so that giving shiatsu is relaxing to do. This is why I have included Section 4 'Do-it-yourself shiatsu' which includes exercises to help you do this. You need to be aware all the time of your working position – how does your back feel, are your hands relaxed? If you work correctly, you will be protecting yourself. You won't get sore thumbs, a bad back or knees. If you are feeling uncomfortable, change your position and re-check how the mother feels. This is an excellent way of getting feedback so that your work is safe. Working with this kind of awareness should encourage you to look after yourself in all areas of your life.

The other aspect of being relaxed is that in essence shiatsu is about 'doing nothing'. This expresses the idea that no effort should be involved; it is about connecting with the mother's energy and allowing change to happen. Sometimes this happens easily, sometimes not so easily, but it is the mother's energy which ultimately decides to change – you cannot make it change. In doing shiatsu we are merely acting as facilitators – it is the other person who is doing the work. We do nothing. In this sense, it is very different from drug-based approaches to healing which put something into the body to make it change. Shiatsu is about working with the energy which is there and in this sense is very safe, as change is limited to what the body can produce and process.

Work from your hara

Shiatsu has its roots in the Eastern traditions of bodywork, which means that it shares similarities with Eastern martial arts. The emphasis in all of these, such as Tai Chi, Qi Qung and karate, is that the centre of the body, the centre of your being, is your hara. The hara covers the area from above your pubic bone, round the side of your body, defined by the anterior iliac spines, to under the rib cage. In some traditions you need to focus on specific points in the hara. An important point is CV-4 – three thumbwidths below the navel, sometimes known as the Dantian.

Working from your hara is the main way in which you can achieve relaxation while you work. It means using your whole body-weight so that individual parts of your body such as your shoulders and hands are not working with effort. The way to cultivate awareness of coming from the hara is by breathing exercises and by movements which encourage the body to move from here.

Exercise 5.1   Hara breathing

Sit in a comfortable position and close your eyes. Begin by noticing how you are breathing now, without altering your breath. Follow the movement of the breath as you breathe out and as you breathe in. Notice which parts of your body move as you breathe. Is your breath fluid? Are you breathing into the hara (abdomen) or is the breath moving more in the rib cage.

Now begin to breathe out more deeply.

Breathe out, for longer, breathe out more slowly. In doing this the breath deepens.

Notice what happens in your hara (abdomen) as you breathe out. Hopefully your abdominal muscles are drawing in, contracting. If this is not the case, try to allow this to happen. It can be helpful to place both hands on your abdomen and try to allow them to be drawn into your body as you breathe out. (You can focus on the point CV-4, three thumbwidths below the navel.)

We say that the out-breath is the Yin breath – the breath of letting go, the breath of relaxation. Our culture emphasizes the in-breath – the Yang aspect of the breath. The in-breath is about taking on new things, drawing things towards us. It is helpful to emphasize the out-breath as this is the aspect of the breath most of us find more difficult to connect with.

As you work with shiatsu, you need to be aware of the breathing of the person you are working with. Often, just placing a hand on someone else and being aware of their out-breath helps them relax and is shiatsu at its simplest level. The Japanese called this 'te ate' which literally means putting a hand on the pain to heal and it is a term often used in nursing practice. All that an experienced shiatsu practitioner knows more is the best place on the body to place the hand, how long to hold it there and how much pressure to give.

Penetrating pressure

At its most basic level, shiatsu is about this kind of energetic contact between you and another person. Try the following exercise.

Exercise 5.2   Back-to-back with a partner (Fig. 5.1)

Sit back-to-back with a partner. Let your whole spine be supported by their spine. Breathe out and lean back into their back. You should feel that you are just resting, just receiving, just feeling support. You should not feel that you are being pushed or are pushing.

With arms linked, try gently rocking from side to side for a few minutes.

With arms linked, try circling. Begin with a small circle and then make the circle bigger. Don't move too quickly. After a while change the direction of the circle.

Then, linking your arms together, one of you can lean as far forward as is comfortable as you both breathe out. Stay in this position for a minute or two, breathing out deeply. Then, on an out-breath, ease back to the upright position for a few breaths. Then the other person can lean forward and you can lean back. Stay in this position for a minute or two breathing out deeply. When you feel ready, as you breathe out, come to the upright position once more.

Feel the differences. What do you feel? Which position did you like best?

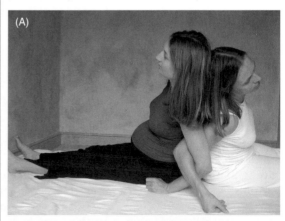
(A)

Figure 5.1   A: Rocking from side to side while sitting back to back.

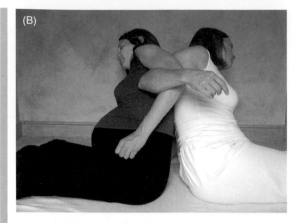

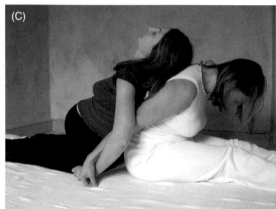

Figure 5.1 *(continued)* B: Rocking from side to side while sitting back to back. C: Leaning forward and backward.

You probably felt as you did this that, by the end, your spine was more relaxed and you may have felt warmth in it. This demonstrates how you can do shiatsu with any part of your body – in this case your back. You give and receive at the same time. Who is giving? Who is receiving? You do nothing other than lean with your body.

Linking hara movements with the use of perpendicular pressure

You need to learn how to integrate breathing from the hara with working with pressure – 'doing something' without doing anything! The simplest way of understanding this idea is to practise some crawling. Crawling is the first way in which we learn to move our body as babies.

Babies live very much from their haras. In going back to this stage of our development, we can learn how to move our bodies naturally, without effort.

Exercise 5.3 Crawling (Fig. 5.2)

Get onto your hands and knees in the all fours position. Breathe out, as in the hara breathing exercise, and throughout try to keep breathing deeply. After a while, rock forwards and backwards and feel your weight shifting from your hands to your knees.

Come to resting.

Now slide your left hand along the ground at the same time as you slide your right knee. When you have gone forwards, move your right hand and left knee. Keep crawling forwards in this way.

As you crawl, imagine that the floor is like someone's back and you are crawling over it. At some point you can try crawling backwards.

Finish by resting in the all fours position.

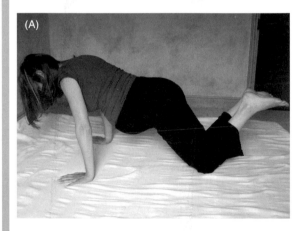

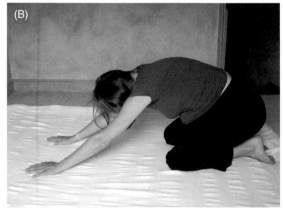

Figure 5.2 A and B: Rocking back and forth on all fours.

When you first start to crawl again, your wrists and knees may begin to hurt. We need to re-learn how to allow our body-weight to be relaxed in our wrists and knees. Many of you probably tell pregnant women to crawl to help get their baby in an optimal position. Yet how often have you tried crawling yourself? It does take time to re-learn it. When you crawl in the way described above, you are integrating left and right brain functions. It is useful in labour to integrate this and, for people of any age, it will help with coordination and balance.

Crawling is the basic position in which we do shiatsu – hands and knees are extensions of the hara. You can use any part of your body to do shiatsu, although for practical reasons we tend mainly to use our hands. It is the weight and energetic connection of the hara behind the hands that provide the connection with the Ki and Essence.

We will now try an exercise to illustrate the way in which we lean our weight into someone else to obtain the type of pressure which we use in shiatsu (see Exercise 5.4).

You should feel that it is much more comfortable to lean your whole body-weight and not try to do anything or hold yourself tensely. You will feel relaxed and less tired. You are not harming your body in any way. It is also more comfortable for the person underneath and feels like a deep, penetrating pressure. When you come from your shoulders, trying to give strong pressure, it is more tiring for you. It is also less comfortable for the person receiving, usually feeling harder, sharper and more invasive.

Being relaxed means feeling comfortable with what you are doing. Throughout the book, when I demonstrate specific points and techniques, you may find that some of the working positions

---

Exercise 5.4   All fours leaning with a partner
(Fig. 5.3)

Get your partner to rest on all fours, either unsupported or leaning over a chair. Lean over them by placing one forearm over their upper back and one over their lower back. Do be careful not to lean your weight in the middle of their back or you could damage it.

Now, lean in a relaxed way, allowing your whole body-weight to rest. Breathe out deeply into your hara as you do this. Stay for a couple of minutes. Now try doing the same but placing your palms on the back.

Now, try the same exercise but rather than relaxing, breathe in, tense your shoulders and feel as though you are trying to apply strong pressure beneath your hands. Please don't actually apply strong pressure as it may well hurt!

How do you feel? How do they respond? Try it both ways round.

This can be a good exercise to give to partners in an antenatal class. It works well as long as there is not a huge difference in weight between the two people doing it. You need to check that people are comfortable before getting them to stay for any length of time. Who is doing the work and who is receiving? This exercise illustrates how shiatsu is about two people's energies working together.

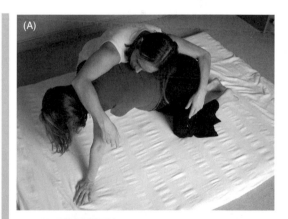

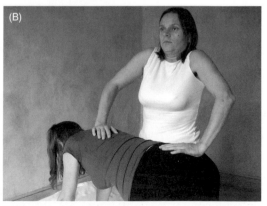

Figure 5.3   Leaning over partner: A, in a relaxed way, allowing the body-weight to rest; and B, incorrectly, note tense shoulders.

are not so comfortable for you, especially if you have an injury. For example, if you have injured your knees then you won't feel comfortable in the crawling positions and may have to adjust your

---

Exercise 5.5 Exploring alternative positions, standing or sitting, and working with static pressure from the hands on the sacrum (Fig. 5.4)

Work with a partner who leans on all fours supported over a chair or birthing ball.

Find a comfortable position in which you can lean from your hara and place one hand on top of the other over your partner's sacrum. Typically, this may be a lunge-type position, with one leg in front of the other. However, if this is uncomfortable, you can try sitting on a chair next to your partner. Have the fingers of your hand which is underneath pointing up the spine and the hand on top laid across at 90°. Let your hands and fingers mould to the shape of your partner's body.

The main point to watch is that, as you lean your body-weight into your hands, you are leaning from your hara. Relax your shoulders and have your elbows slightly bent – but don't bend your arms too much otherwise you won't be applying any pressure and you keep leaning in more to no effect. Don't look down with your head because that tends to round your upper back. It is your hands and hara doing the work – not your head. Gently begin to experiment with different pressures on your partner's sacral area and also experiment with moving your hands up and down the sacrum. Remember to keep breathing out and working from your hara.

Get feedback from your partner as to how much pressure feels comfortable and how long you need to stay in different areas.

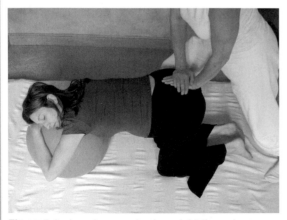

Figure 5.4 Leaning your body-weight through your palms into the sacrum.

positions. That is fine. Remember that shiatsu was developed originally in Japan, where people were used to kneeling. Their hips and legs were flexible. However, today, even many Japanese are not as comfortable in their traditional sitting positions since they are more used to sitting in chairs and driving cars. The main principle is that the movement of your body comes from your hara. This means that you need to face the area you are working and keep your hips relaxed and open so you can lean forward without twisting. Your arms and shoulders also need to be relaxed. You can apply this principle in any position, as in Exercise 5.5.

Stationary pressure is usually experienced as deeply relaxing. It works on the parasympathetic nervous system which, in turn, calms the internal organs and the body as a whole. The amount of pressure you need to use will depend to some extent on the part of the body you are working. The sacrum can take quite strong pressure; by contrast the neck needs much lighter pressure. It also depends on the person you are working on. Some people like strong pressure, others less. Generally, bigger people prefer stronger pressure, babies less. Always remember it is not a physical effort, it is relaxing, penetrating pressure, which goes deep in the body to connect with its basic energies.

Work to balance Kyo and Jitsu

As shiatsu is about balancing energy in the body, the way in which we work is determined by the condition of the energy which we feel. There are the two 'opposite' types of energy defined by Kyo and Jitsu. These concepts are very similar to Yin and Yang, but refer to unhealthy expressions of energy:

- Kyo is the condition of *depleted energy*, which is more *hypo*.
- Jitsu is the condition of *excess energy*, which is more *hyper*.

Masunaga liked to use the illustration of thinking of a round ball representing a healthy person (Masunaga 1977). Now think of a distorted ball with indentations and protrusions around it. The indentations are hollow and represent Kyo. The protrusions are Jitsu. This idea represents the concept of the whole energy being connected – the ball is like the Tao. If one area is protruding, there must be another area which is indented. It is easier to spot the Jitsu areas because they project from the surface, but it is much more difficult to find the Kyo areas which are hidden. In shiatsu we say that the 'problem' is the Jitsu, but the 'cause' is the Kyo. We spend time first working with the Kyo and bringing energy to it. This energy has to come from somewhere where there is too much energy – the Jitsu area. Sometimes this is enough, sometimes we need to then work directly on the Jitsu area, moving energy away from it.

Another way of thinking of this is to consider the example of a pregnant woman who has tight shoulders and a tense jaw. The jaw is where she perceives the problem to be. As you may remember from Section 2, this is often linked with wood energy being stuck, perhaps as a result of lack of physical activity, worry or frustration. We observe that she has a weak and cold lower back and begin to work here first. This is the Kyo area. If we first worked her shoulders, it could be very

painful and difficult to release. By working on her back, energy is drawn down from the shoulders, without us even working here directly. After this, when we go to the shoulders, they are already softer and respond well (Fig. 5.5).

You may think that it is hard to learn to see and feel Kyo and Jitsu – but remember it is a very instinctive reaction. Often we notice someone's stiff shoulders and want to work with them, but it may be painful so we place a hand somewhere else on the body.

Most people find it quite easy to spot these two qualities of energy and even to feel them balancing out, simply by holding the hands over the two areas. The body naturally wants to balance out these two extremes of energy. This is all that a shiatsu practitioner is doing in their work – finding the most Kyo area in the body and bringing energy to it, and finding the most Jitsu area and allowing energy to flow from it. A shiatsu practitioner will be able to identify which meridian they are on and if they are on a particular point. In a sense that identification isn't as important as the act of balancing Kyo and Jitsu, and helping the body to come to more of a sense of balance.

Exercise 5.6   To feel Kyo and Jitsu

Get someone to sit in front of you. Close your eyes and focus on breathing from your hara. When you are relaxed, open your eyes but have them slightly out of focus. Look at your partner's back. See if you can notice any areas where you feel there is a lot of active energy – we could call this tension. Now try to look for areas where you feel that there is not much going on, areas where there is a weakness or depletion with not enough energy.

Now place one of your hands over the area where you feel there is not much going on. Don't apply pressure, just make contact with the area. Feel the quality of what is beneath your hand.

Now place the other hand over the full area whilst keeping the first hand over the Kyo area. What do you feel on this full or Jitsu area?

Now focus on the connection between your two hands. Try to imagine that the energy is flowing from the full area to the empty area. Keep your hands over the two areas until you feel there is some more balance, less of a difference between the two. You may even feel that they are the same by the end.

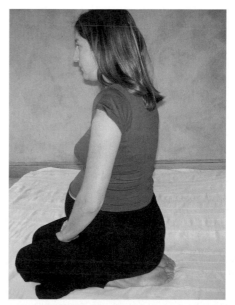

Figure 5.5   A woman with Jitsu (tense) shoulders and Kyo (weak) lower back.

Table 5.1 There are many qualities associated with Kyo and Jitsu. Which of the following qualities did you feel when you did the exercise?

Kyo	Jitsu
Empty	Full
Expansion	Contraction
Loose/flaccid	Tight
Deep	Surface
Slow	Fast
Cold	Hot
Yielding	Resisting
Weak	Strong
Soft	Hard
Depleted	Energetic
Receptive	Repellent
Drawing in	Pushing away
Muscle – atrophied, underused	Muscle – hypertonic, over-used

Table 5.2 Ways of working with Kyo and Jitsu – tonification and dispersion

Tonifying techniques for Kyo	Sedating/dispersing techniques for Jitsu
Hold for longer – generally more emphasis on holding techniques	Hold for less – generally more emphasis on movement and stretches
Use soft parts of your body e.g. palm	Use sharper parts of your body e.g. elbow
Use slow stroking techniques	Use faster stroking techniques
Work more slowly	Work more quickly
Work with the aim to bring energy towards	Work with the aim of moving energy away

Although simply by holding the two points change can occur, in shiatsu we tend to use different techniques with the Kyo and Jitsu areas. This is something which is instinctive. The Kyo area naturally draws you into it. You will tend to want to stay longer, to hold the areas, to use long, slow and soft strokes. Your focus with the Kyo areas is to nurture, to strengthen and bring energy to them. This is known as *tonification*.

With the Jitsu areas you will naturally want to move energy away; you will tend to want to use shorter, sharper, faster strokes, maybe even some stretches. These types of techniques are called *sedation/dispersion*.

Like with Yin and Yang, these are relative concepts. In some people there may not be big differences between the Kyo and Jitsu. With others, there may be huge variations. With some people, you may have a strong sense that overall their energy is Kyo, and you need to work more with tonifying techniques. With other people you may feel that overall their energy is more Jitsu, and you may need to work more with sedating techniques. This relates to some people being more Yang and others more Yin. Pregnancy is more Yin than labour which is more Yang, and so in labour we tend to work more with sedating techniques and in pregnancy with more tonifying techniques.

The person giving shiatsu needs to know when energy is Jitsu or Kyo or when it is simply full and empty. This is where a midwife trained in shiatsu skills may have an advantage over a shiatsu practitioner without midwifery knowledge. In pregnancy the hara feels full because it contains the developing baby. This fullness is not Jitsu – it needs to be there. An inexperienced practitioner may mistakenly try to move the 'Jitsu' from the hara. This would be unsafe in the first trimester when the energies of the baby and placenta are forming. Later on in pregnancy, this fullness in the hara may indeed have Jitsu qualities, for example the mother may feel pressure under her ribs or in the groin. Now that the baby's energy is stable, some appropriate sedating work may need to be done to help the mother and baby feel more space. In labour, the full energy of the uterus needs to move the baby and placenta down to the perineum. This powerful energy needs to be supported if it gets blocked – either with tonifying or sedating techniques. We need to remember that, like Yin and Yang, Kyo and Jitsu are not static. The body's energies are constantly changing. With a good understanding of the processes of the body, it is easy to know where to move the energies to.

Ultimately, working against the body's energy will not feel right – although, as every midwife knows, so much is happening in pregnancy that a mother may not know what is meant to be going on. Shiatsu in the maternity period is about enabling women to be more aware of what is going on in their body. I wonder if this is why many shiatsu practitioners have been wary of working with pregnancy. It is not safe to work in pregnancy unless the practitioner has a good understanding of what is meant to be happening. Midwives do and therefore, with proper shiatsu training, it is safe for them to do shiatsu in the maternity period.

How long do I need to stay?

Remember what you felt with two hands holding Kyo and Jitsu areas. At some point, you may have felt a balancing between the two, or maybe you just felt less of a difference – the Kyo felt fuller, the Jitsu felt less tight. It is this type of change we are looking for with shiatsu, and it is hard to quantify how much change it can be, because it varies from person to person and from situation to situation. You will find with practice you develop a sense of how long to stay. The mother will also be able to tell you. If you have stayed for too long, it no longer feels as comfortable. While you are beginning to do shiatsu you will find that you need to get lots of feedback from the people you are working on. They will be able to tell you what feels good and what doesn't feel so good. As long as you follow them and the basic principles, your work will not only be safe, but also fairly effective. Shiatsu is not about holding points and counting to a number. An instruction such as 'hold the point for 20 s every half an hour during labour' has no meaning with shiatsu. This time could be too long for one person and not long enough for another.

So far, we have only looked at holding techniques which tend to be more for Kyo areas. Now we will look at stroking techniques which tend to be more dispersing, but used slowly can also be tonifying.

Exercise 5.7 Stroking exercise (Fig. 5.6)

Get your partner to lean over a chair in the all fours position. Place your two hands anywhere on the top of their back and allow them to rest without applying pressure. Make sure that you are comfortable and working from your hara. Begin to stroke lightly down the back with a continuous, hand over hand movement. Move slowly to start with and cover the whole back, including the spine and the buttocks. Now, gradually speed up the stroking for a while. After a while increase the pressure slightly so it is firmer. After a while use the firmer pressure with

slower strokes. Gradually, move down over the buttocks to the legs, working one leg at a time. Finish by holding the foot for a minute or so. It is important to allow the energy to settle at the end.

You can try the stroking with your partner in other positions such as sitting, lying on their side or even standing. Make sure that you adjust your working position accordingly.

Swap over with your partner, so you feel this yourself.

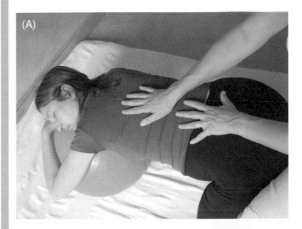

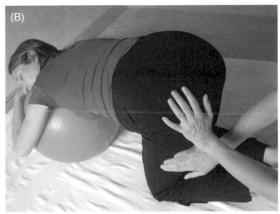

Figure 5.6 Stroking: A, over the back; and B, down the buttocks.

What did you feel about the different strokes? Some people prefer one of the strokes, some like some strokes over some areas and other strokes over different areas. This shows differences with Kyo and Jitsu areas in the body. The more Kyo areas need holding or slower, deeper strokes. The more Jitsu areas need faster, lighter stroking to move the energy away.

You will have noticed that I included stroking over the spine. In shiatsu, the spine is considered to be very important and we work directly with it, like osteopaths, chiropractors and yoga teachers. Some of you who may have done massage training may have been told not to work on the spine – this is a caution for basic massage work for people without a thorough understanding of anatomy. In order to work on the spine, you need to be aware of how much pressure is suitable, as well as precautions such as not working with herniated discs.

Work with two hands – work with continuity and flow

One of the key features of working with shiatsu, which is slightly different from working with massage, is the technique of working with two hands. This is following the Kyo–Jitsu principle, in which one hand assumes a supportive, or Yin role, and the other hand an active, or Yang role. The Yin hand is known as the 'mother hand'. This tends to be still while the other hand, the 'working hand' moves round the body. By working with these two forces at the same time, we can promote balanced energy in the body. The supportive or Yin hand is very important – it provides the penetrating support needed to prepare the body for shiatsu. Without this force, the manipulation with the hand in motion (Yang) will remain superficial and often painful.

Exercise 5.8   To feel the mother hand and working hand, and to work using palming and thumb pressures (Figs 5.7, 5.8)

Have your partner resting on all fours. Place one hand on their upper back and one hand on their lower back. It doesn't matter where your hands are positioned exactly, because the aim of this is to make an initial contact with your partner and to see if you can feel their breathing. Allow your hands to rest lightly. Ask your partner to breathe out deeply, maybe making a sound as she breathes out.

Check that your position is comfortable, your wrists and elbows are relaxed and you are breathing from your hara.

Stay for a few minutes and see how much you can feel your partner's breathing through your hands. If your partner asks you to move your hand position slightly so it is more comfortable, do so.

Now place one hand on an area of the back you feel is Kyo. If you're not sure just place it anywhere – this hand is going to remain still and will be the mother hand. Place the other hand on the top right side of the back – this is the working hand. As your partner breathes out, lean in, applying some pressure with both hands. Feel how much pressure to apply and see if you can feel a connection with both hands. Never apply more pressure with the working hand than with the mother hand. Try to see if you can feel a flow of energy between the two hands.

Stay as long as you feel you need – you may feel a shift like you felt when you worked holding Kyo and Jitsu. If you're not sure how long to stay, stay for about three to four of your partner's out-breaths.

When you feel that you have stayed long enough, slide your working hand a little way down the right side of the back, keeping the mother hand still. Allow the working hand to mould to the shape of the mother's body and feel the weight of your body going through the centre of your palm. See if you can get a sense of how long to stay in this new place – but stay at least for a couple of the mother's out-breaths. You may feel that with each out-breath you feel a shift of energy. Experiment with different pressures. After you feel you have stayed long enough in this new place, slide the working hand down again a short way and repeat the process. This is the technique I refer to as *palming*.

As you move your working hand, if you need to change your body's position so that you are leaning and breathing from you hara, do so.

Repeat this, but using the thumb pad of the working hand. This is the technique I refer to as *thumb pressure*. When you have palmed down the right side of the back, do the same down the left side of the back.

Now, place the mother hand over the sacrum and, with the working hand, palm down the back of the legs. When you reach the knee, move your mother hand and place it above the knee and palm down the lower leg with the working hand.

Repeat this, but using the thumb pad of the working hand.

As you work, make sure that you lean in from your hara. Make sure the pressure is angled at 90° to the mother's body.

Get a sense of how strong the pressure is in each place and how long you need to stay. Can you feel different textures beneath your two hands? Can you feel a connection between the two hands?

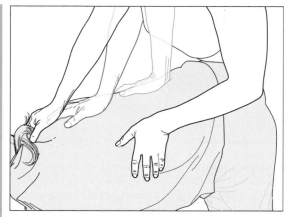

Figure 5.7 Palming down the back.

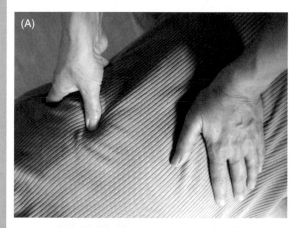

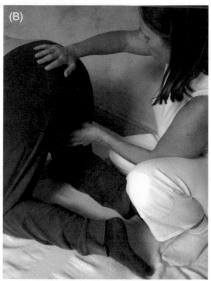

Figure 5.8 A: Working with thumb pressures down the back. B: Using thumb pressure down the leg.

By working with two hands, we are working on the areas beneath each hand as well as the area between them. The two hands need to be close enough so that as you lean you can feel that you are leaning from your hara into both hands. When they are too far apart and you feel that you are over-stretching, simply move the mother hand and find another place to put it. If you can identify a Kyo area it is usually best to place the mother hand here.

Think of the mother hand as being like a plug into the body's energy. If we only have one hand in contact, then we do not provide a circuit. When we do stroking movements, we don't have the mother hand, but we still need to provide a continuous movement otherwise we break contact with the energy. When we use two hands on one place (like in the sacral exercise) we can say that the hand underneath is the working hand and the hand on top is the mother hand. If we work with the thumbs of the two hands, then the rest of the hand needs to act as the mother hand, both to support your thumbs and the energy of the other person.

Case study 5.1   Sheila, community midwife in London

Being a midwife involves being 'with woman' as every midwife and woman in labour knows. I was privileged to be taught by some experienced and gifted midwives who gave so much to the women in their care. I learnt how touch, massage and applying pressure can provide so much relief for women in labour and showed any interested birth partners how they could assist and be involved. However, I often found this quite exhausting. One of the major things that shiatsu has in its favour is that it does not deplete the energy of the practitioner and in fact may enhance it.

Working through the clothes or using oils

Shiatsu was always traditionally done through the clothes and most shiatsu practitioners continue this tradition. The idea behind this is that the energy that we are touching does not just relate to the skin and the muscle but to something deep in the core of the body, the meridians, basic

Ki, life-force and Essence. It was also probably a cultural tradition which developed in Japan from the point of view of modesty. For some people, one of the attractions of shiatsu is that the recipient can remain fully clothed, and many pregnant women and new mothers will find this more acceptable. In a class situation it is less threatening for people to learn techniques whilst fully clothed, especially if they have not done any kind of bodywork before. However, you don't have to be that rigid. There are some traditions of shiatsu where work is done directly on the skin using oil. During labour, the mother may not be wearing clothes and this doesn't mean that shiatsu cannot be done.

If you are going to use oil, then it is best to use cold-pressed or organic wherever possible. Most vegetable oils are suitable. You can buy these from your local supermarket or healthfood shop – a good guide is if you can eat it, it's probably going to be alright to put on your skin. Don't use mineral oils, i.e. liquidium parafinnum, as they can deplete the skin of vitamins A and D. Almond oil was often used traditionally, but there is now an increased incidence of allergies (although still rare; nut allergies tend to be more related to peanuts) – so use with caution. Do a patch test first – see baby section below. You can use other vegetable oils like sunflower, safflower, grape-seed, coconut oil or castor oil. These plain vegetable oils are known as the base oil.

In pregnancy, wheat-germ oil or evening primrose which are high in vitamin E can be mixed in a ratio of 25% to 75% of a vegetable base oil. Vitamin E may also be used – you can buy a capsule of this and break it into the base oil you are going to use. All these oils may help minimize stretch marks on the abdomen, although remember that these are the result of overstretching of the skin and are ultimately dependent on the mother's weight gain and skin structure. The mother may also want to use them to nourish the skin of the perineum to help it stretch during the birth.

In labour, it is best to keep to the same oils used during pregnancy. Postnatally, in Japan, white sesame oil was used for shiatsu on the breasts, which was done directly on the skin. A discussion of aromatherapy oils is beyond the scope of this book, although there are some traditions of shiatsu which link particular oils to particular meridians. It is important to remember that these are medicinal oils and should only be used in conjunction with a qualified aromatherapist.

For the baby

Shiatsu for the baby depends on the situation. If the mother has little time, or the weather is cold (winters in some areas of Japan are very cold), then shiatsu can be done through the clothes. If the mother has more time and the weather is warm or the room heated, shiatsu can be done with oil directly on the skin. There is no need to use any oils in the first few days, unless the baby's skin is dry. A soft touch alone is beneficial. Make sure that whichever oil is going to be used is tested on a small area of the baby's skin first and then, if there is no allergic reaction within 24 h, repeat again. If there is still no allergic reaction after a further 24 h, then you can use the oil. The same kind of oils which are suitable for mothers are also suitable for babies. Use almond oil with caution. Olive oil is excellent for cradle cap and also patches of dry skin, but is rather heavy and smelly to use over the whole body. Other vegetable oils are also suitable, particularly apricot kernel, peach kernel, fractionated coconut and grape-seed. With a baby, it is preferable to use organic, cold-pressed oils if possible, especially on babies with sensitive skins.

Summary

The essence of shiatsu is about a simple way of touching the body based on a view of looking at the body as an energy field. At this level it is safe to do and incorporates easily into existing midwifery practices. You may find many of these basic techniques are similar to some of what you do instinctively. Remember that shiatsu developed out of people working on the body. It began with practical applications and then theory was evolved to explain the practice.

Reflect on the following questions:

- What are the similarities and differences between shiatsu and other forms of bodywork such as massage, reflexology and aromatherapy?
- What do you think falls within your scope of practice?
- What do you feel you have already been doing instinctively?
- What are you not doing?
- Which concepts are new to you?
- Do you have difficulty understanding any of these concepts? If so, identify which and go back to try to see what you don't understand.
- What could you begin to incorporate into your practice and how?

REFERENCES

Masunaga S 1977 Zen shiatsu. Japan Publications, Tokyo

Pitchford P 1993 Healing through whole foods. North Atlantic Books, Berkeley, California

FURTHER READING

Lundberg P 1973 The book of shiatsu. Gaia Books, London

Jarmey C, Mojay G 1999 Shiatsu – the complete guide. Thorsons, London

Kusmirek J 2002 Liquid sunshine – vegetable oils for aromatherapy. Floramicus, Somerset

Meeus C 2001 Secrets of shiatsu. Dorling Kindersley, London

Pooley N 1998 Shiatsu in a nutshell. Element Books, Shaftesbury, Dorset

6

Shiatsu for labour

Introduction

In a sense, working with a woman in labour is one of the easiest times to do shiatsu. A woman in labour is extremely sensitive to the kind of touch she needs and where she needs it. You may find some of what follows is similar to what you already do; shiatsu is simply giving you more of an awareness of why you do what you do, and offering a tool to deepen the quality of your work. A midwife trained in shiatsu skills may not work that differently from an experienced shiatsu practitioner, as working in labour is about seeing where to move the energy. Midwives are often able to see that as easily as a shiatsu practitioner as they are very in tune with the energies of labour.

Work in labour may involve strong, often dispersing, techniques as the energy is so intense and powerful. The focus is on helping the body's energies to flow well right from the beginning, rather than waiting till they get stuck, when it is much harder to change the patterns. In terms of shiatsu for 'pain relief', we can say that the body feels less pain or is able to cope better with pain if it is being supported to do what it needs to do. Indeed, both traditionally and even today in Japan, women are just expected to get on with labour and, not surprisingly, with that expectation, they often do. In shiatsu, we are not trying to take away the pain, but enable the mother to work with her body. From this point of view, it is useful to involve both the mother and her birth partner even before labour. Introducing shiatsu in antenatal classes enables them both to approach labour more positively and to feel that there is something that they can do. Parents can be taught induction points as long as they are taught to work with feedback from the mother, so that if it doesn't feel right, then they discontinue until they have re-checked with the midwife. It is, however, never too late to begin shiatsu. Even in the second stage women can respond positively.

Remember that how points and meridians are touched is as important as locating the correct position of a point. Be aware of the mother's breathing and try to apply or increase pressure as she breathes out. It may be helpful for you to breathe with her and then this also becomes a way of supporting her to breathe more deeply. Often points are stimulated during contractions, the amount of pressure increasing as the intensity of contractions increases. In between stimulating the points, it may be relaxing for both you and the mother for you to do some stroking movements, either light or vigorous, or to apply lighter general pressure.

Many techniques are useful for different stages of labour, but eventually you will be able to select which one is most suitable for the energy of the particular woman you are working with. You need to try to tune into Kyo and Jitsu, and decide where the mother has too much energy and where she doesn't have enough.

I don't give specific times for how long to work a point or a meridian because shiatsu is about responding to the individual. Some people are more sensitive and may feel a strong reaction after a few seconds. Other people may not feel very much, even after a few minutes. However, labour is a time when points may be held for much longer than usual. In pregnancy and postnatally, or if you are practising with friends, a few minutes is often long enough. In labour, by contrast, some of the points may need to be worked on for hours. If a mother finds a particular point helpful, she may not want you to stop. In this case, it is useful to enlist the support of her partner, so you can attend to your other duties! It is the same with shiatsu for induction. If a woman is not going into labour, then sometimes working once with the induction points for a few minutes may be enough to stimulate contractions, but it may be that the points need to be worked for up to an hour several times a day for

several days. Sometimes I get women to stick a grain of rice on the point with a plaster and stimulate as often as they feel is right through the day. The guideline I give for induction is to work the points as often and for as long as it feels right. The mother usually feels something – whether it be relaxation or movement of the baby or a contraction itself. She knows how long she needs the point to be stimulated and which is the most effective one.

I present most versions of the techniques with the mother in the all fours position. By this, I mean on her hands and knees leaning over a chair, as this is a good position for supporting the process of birth. The work is the same if the mother is sitting astride a chair, leaning against the wall or kneeling forwards. You are still able to access the same parts of the body. You need to make sure that the pressures are appropriate for the position in which you are working. You can also do shiatsu with the mother lying on her side or back, or indeed any position, as long as you apply the basic principles. I will focus more on how to work in these two other positions in the pregnancy and postnatal sections and you can refer to these for more guidance on this.

I have included some visualizations on each of the different elements. These can sometimes be useful for the mother to focus on in labour and they can be introduced during antenatal classes. They can also be helpful to do as a midwife, to be more aware of the energy of the different meridians.

Back routines

The back is important to work in labour because the spine relates to Governing Vessel energy which is the main source of Yang energy and which regulates Essence and Ki in the body. The Bladder meridian passes down each side of the spine and this part of the Bladder meridian contains points that relate to all the organs in the body – the Yu or associated organ points (Fig. 6.1). Bladder also relates to the nervous system. We can say that by working on the back we are able to balance all energies in the body. Water energy (Bladder) is especially important in the first stage when fear can block the process of labour. The spine

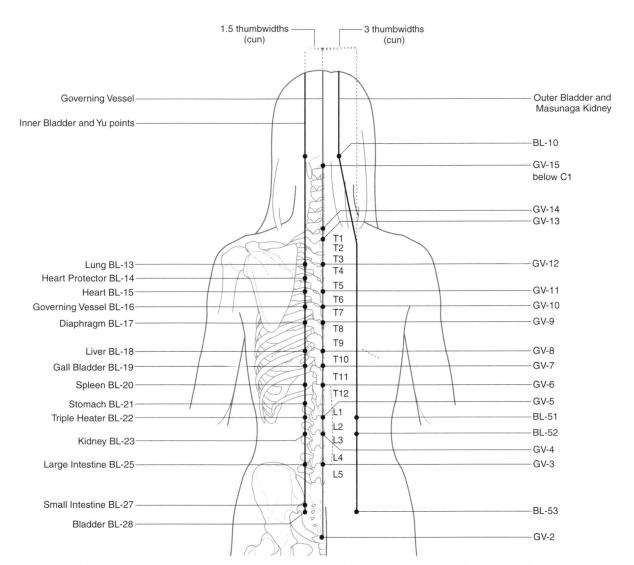

Figure 6.1 The main meridians of the back – Kidney, Bladder and Governing Vessel – and important points including Yu points. Note: remember all meridians are bi-lateral.

provides the main physical and emotional support for the body and is an area where tension can be stored in labour. The sacrum and neck can be areas where the mother may experience discomfort.

I have included Fig. 6.1 so you can see the different points, but you don't necessarily need to learn where they all are, unless you are a shiatsu practitioner. You may become familiar with some of the important ones such as BL-21 (Stomach), BL-20 (Spleen), BL-22 (Triple Heater and lower burner, fluids), BL-23 (Kidney). All the associated points are in a line one and a half thumbwidths from the midline of the spine. A thumbwidth or

cun is the measurement the Japanese/Chinese used to measure the location of points. It is one thumbwidth of the person that you are working on and not your own. You need to remember this especially when you are working with a baby.

Other important points are:

- BL-51. This is level with BL-22 on the back, three thumbwidths from the midline, and it affects the Triple Heater. The Ki of the Triple Heater is essential for the proper movement and transportation of Ki in all physiological processes. Its action extends up to the chest and downwards to the Bladder and Uterus.

It is used in postpartum abdominal pain, breast lumps and breast pain.

- Jinggong (Palace of the Essence). This coincides with BL-52, i.e. three thumbwidths from the midline, level with BL-23; it tonifies the Kidneys and Essence.
- BL-53. This is level with the spinous process of the second sacral vertebra, three thumbwidths from the midline. Its action affects the abdomen, bladder, uterus and genitals.
- GV-4 is an important point in regulating the fire of the Kidneys (Ming Men). It also clears heat, regulates the GV, tonifies the Kidneys and benefits the lumbar spine.

It is helpful to know what the points are for, but what is most important is to balance Kyo and Jitsu along the meridian lines – if you do this, you will be balancing energy appropriately. Ikuyo Hosaka used these back points a lot in her work, but didn't always seem to name the actions of the points.

Before you work on the Bladder meridian, I'd like you to connect with the energy of water. This can be useful for women as preparation for labour and can be used in labour itself. It illustrates how instinctive shiatsu is – as many women naturally feel an affinity with the image of the wave, or indeed even want to be in water during their labour.

Box 6.1   Water visualizations

With all the visualizations, find a comfortable position in which to do them. This could be lying, sitting or resting on all fours, or indeed any position.

The wave

The wave is a familiar image women tune into in labour – because it links into the water energy. The wave allows us to contact the Yang, dynamic, moving aspects of water. This wave visualization can be done either in pregnancy or in labour itself.

Sit and close your eyes.

Follow the movement of breath as you breathe out and in. As you breathe out, lengthen the breath and allow it to drop into the abdomen (hara) so as you breathe out your abdominal muscles gently draw in.

After a short while, as you breathe out, imagine that the breath is like a wave of water moving through your body.

You can feel it spreading out from your hara to cover your whole body from head to toe.

You can feel the wave beginning at the top of your head and allow it to flow down through your whole body.

Keep focusing on your out-breath as you feel it flowing down the outside – from your head, over your shoulders and back and down over your chest and ribs into the pelvis. Feel it flowing down the pelvis and then over the buttocks and abdomen and into the legs. Feel it flowing down your legs into your feet. Feel it flowing out from the soles of your feet.

Keep focusing on your out-breath as you feel it flowing down the inside of your body. Focus on your main organs. Feel it flowing through your nose as your breathe out and in. Feel it flowing through your lungs as they expand and empty. Feel it flowing through your heart as it beats. Feel it flowing through your intestines as water cleansing. Feel it flowing through your uterus and surrounding your baby. Be aware of it flowing around your baby's body. Feel it flowing through your cervix. In labour, the mother can feel it flowing in the cervix and opening it out, but do not suggest doing this in pregnancy.

Ease out when you feel ready.

The pool

The lake enables us to contact the Yin, still, supportive aspect of water.

Breathe out deeply into the hara.

When you feel relaxed, imagine that you are lying in a pool of warm water. You feel the water supporting your body so that you do not have to do anything except lie back and relax. With each out-breath feel a deeper sense of peace and support.

Be aware of your baby in the pool with you. Your baby may be in their own pool of water inside you, the water of the amniotic sac. Or maybe they are lying in the pool of water next to you or lying on your abdomen. As you breathe out feel yourself floating with your baby. Sense how your baby's body is supported by the water.

Ease out when you feel ready.

Basic techniques

With all these techniques, start working with the mother in the all fours position lying over a chair. When you are familiar with them, you can work with the mother in any position.

Make sure that you apply all the basic principles previously presented, especially remembering to move and breathe from your hara.

Coccyx release

Contact the left side of the upper cervical vertebrae, i.e. just under below the occiput, with the fingertips of one hand, and the left side of the coccyx with the fingertips of the other. Feel which is more Kyo and which is more Jitsu. Imagine a flow of energy between them, and see if a subtle rocking motion occurs. If it does, move your hands in time with it, accentuating the flow. If not, apply pressure alternatively for as long as you feel appropriate. Repeat this on the other side and then in the midline with the upper fingers in the central indentation at the base of the occiput, and the lower fingers on the coccyx. Repeat with two fingers applying pressure on either side of the coccyx at the same time (Fig. 6.2). Release may be felt as a tingling, warmth, or a spreading out.

Occipito-sacral rocking/balance

Do the same as you did for the coccyx release, but this time cup the occiput with one hand and place the palm of the other over the sacrum (Fig. 6.3). Respond to any rhythm you may feel.

Why? You are making a connection with the spinal column and the cerebrospinal fluid which is the energy of the Governing Vessel meridian. This runs right through the spinal column, and some important points (GV-15 and GV-2) may be underneath your hands. The coccyx is an important area on the Governing Vessel. If energy is blocked here then there can be lower backache or blockages in the process of labour, especially in second stage when the coccyx needs to move. The sacrum also relates to Bladder energy and to the flow of Essence and the Governing Vessel. Both holds can be useful if the mother is very exhausted at any stage of labour – if she has a depletion of Yang energy. If the Yang energy of the mother is too active then the neocortex will be over-stimulated and she may be frightened. The hold may quieten the energy, or it may be that you need to do some more dispersing-type work such as faster palming or stroking.

Palming and using thumb pressure on the Governing Vessel, Kidney and Bladder

You can very gently palm down the Governing Vessel, keeping your mother hand over the coccyx, or moving it slightly higher, as feels appropriate. Refer back to the basic techniques on pages 82–83 for a description of palming. Begin with your working hand at the neck and work down to the coccyx. You need to use light holding on the neck and also in the middle of the back, because strong pressure in this position could damage this part of the spine. Remember to keep the mother hand–working hand connection.

Now that we are palming on a specific meridian, unlike the general palming previously described, you need to focus your attention on getting the centre of your palm over the centre of the meridian being worked – in this case the centre of the spine. Still remember to mould your whole hand to the mother's body. You also need to make sure that you are leaning your body-weight in at 90° to the angle of her body so that the pressure penetrates deep inside. You can tell if you are not doing this because often you will find you are pulling up or down on skin or clothes. You may even move the mother's body.

As you palm, see if you can notice the more Kyo and the more Jitsu areas. Repeat this as often as is comfortable – sense how long you need to stay on each area.

You can also palm with the centre of your palm over a line 1.5 thumbwidths out from the

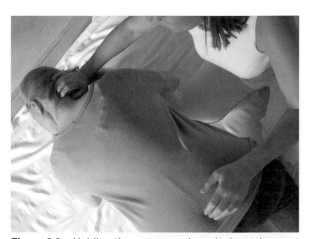

Figure 6.2 Holding the coccyx and cervical vertebrae.

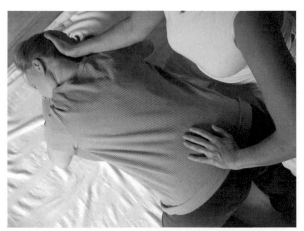

Figure 6.3 Balancing occipital and sacral energies.

midline of the spine which we locate as the highest point of the erectae spinae muscles. This is working the traditional Bladder meridian.

You can palm out 3 thumbwidths from the midline of the spine – this is working the Masunaga extended Kidney meridian.

It is usually best to palm down these meridians, i.e. from the neck to the sacrum, rather than upwards, from the sacrum to the neck, as the focus in labour is to bring energy into the uterus, abdomen and lower back areas. If there is a reason to bring energy away from these areas such as precipitate labour or hypertonic contractions then you can work in the other direction.

You can repeat work with these meridians using your thumb pads instead of your palms, as in the basic techniques.

Why? All these meridians are important in labour. Bladder and Kidney represent the water element which is drawn upon a lot in labour – they can be used any time the mother is feeling tired or exhausted. If you feel she is stuck, either physically or emotionally, then working with these may promote a sense of flow and movement. This may also affect the baby, either through promoting movement or calming. They may help with urination. As the emotion of water is fear, they can be used whenever there is fear.

The Bladder meridian extends from the eye, over the head, down the back and to the feet. Because of its length, it has a great range of actions which are not just limited to the Bladder organ and it is one of the most important meridians in the body. It includes the Yu points in the back which affect all the other organs in the body. (Bladder is useful for backache in labour.) The Governing Vessel regulates Yang, Ki and Essence (see above). Palming slowly is more tonifiying, palming more quickly is more dispersing/sedating.

Hand-over-hand stroking

You can use the stroking technique over the back, neck and shoulders – moving hand over hand and working from the top down, like we did in the basic technique section, but this time focusing more specifically on the meridians of GV/BL/KI. The direction is important as it is more relaxing this way and draws tension away from the neck and shoulders. Make sure that your wrists and shoulders are relaxed and have your whole hand in contact with the body. You can work lightly over the neck, more firmly over the shoulders, more lightly down the spine and quite firmly down the legs. You may want to finish off holding the feet.

Experiment with a colleague to feel the effects of different speeds – go as slowly as you can and as quickly as you can and everything in between. If you do it more slowly it is more relaxing and is more about bringing energy into the Kyo areas. If you do it quickly, it is more stimulating and sedates the Jitsu areas.

Why? This is a deeply relaxing stroke and can be used at any time in labour when you want to support the mother to relax and let go, and for the same reasons as you would palm these meridians.

All three techniques can potentially be used at any stage of labour – but they are especially helpful between first-stage contractions to help the mother to fully use the space to relax and let go of the pain of the previous contraction and be ready for the next contraction. They can also help her to regain her energy, so can be useful if she is tired. They help her feel more in touch with herself and can help her to feel less anxious. This can also apply to the transition between the contractions of first and second stage, and indeed between second and third stage if there is a delayed physiological delivery of the placenta.

Decide if the woman seems more Yin or more Yang and if her energies feel more Kyo or Jitsu to judge whether to use the more holding techniques (i.e. tonification) or the more stimulating techniques (i.e. sedation).

Stronger pressure on the sacrum

It is possible to give much stronger pressure on the sacrum. Review this basic technique, including Fig. 5.4, from p. 78. Begin by placing one hand on top of the other in a criss-cross pattern, the fingers of the lower hand facing up the spine. Begin at the top of the sacrum, i.e. just below the level of the iliac crests, and palm down to over the coccyx. Repeat this a few times, gradually building up to the maximum pressure which is comfortable for the mother as you do so. Make sure that the pressure applied is at an angle of 90° to the mother's body and keep remembering to work and breathe from your hara.

You can apply pressure into each buttock. You can have one hand on each buttock and angle the pressure at 90° to the body in both hands equally at the same time, but making sure that you feel a connection between the two hands.

Why? In labour, the mother often feels tightness, pressure or pain in the sacrum. She may feel the pain of the contractions directly in this area, a pain which often spreads down the legs. This relates to the water energy in the body. With pressure this pain can be eased.

The sacrum is also related to the neck – tension in the neck can often be expressed in the sacrum. Sometimes the neck can be too painful to work on directly, so work on the sacrum is useful. The same holds true the other way round – thus work on the neck may be indicated if pressure on the sacrum is too strong.

The sacrum forms part of the structure of the pelvis, and, by working on it, all other joints in the pelvis may be affected such as the sacro-iliac joint and the symphysis pubis; thus it can be used to ease pain in these joints as well.

More complex techniques

Sacral opening/gathering

Sacral opening You can apply pressure to each side of the sacrum. To release energy from the sacrum and send it to the front, place your hands so that your fingers are pointing out, and align the heels of the hands along the outer edge of the sacrum. Lean both hands in at 90° but with a slight opening to the sides of the body so that you open up the sides of the sacrum (Fig. 6.4A).

Sacral gathering The opposite of this is to place your hands so that your fingers are pointing to the centre, with the heel of the hand still along the outer edge of the sacrum. Your hands may overlap. As the mother breathes out, lean both hands in at 90°, at the same time slightly drawing them together. This brings energy into the sacrum and opens it up around the symphysis pubis. Do not do this strongly if the mother is

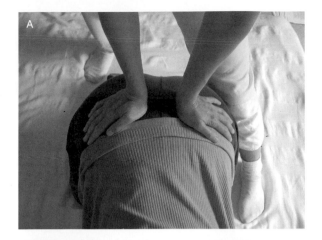

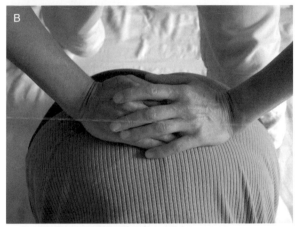

Figure 6.4 A: Sacral opening and B: sacral gathering.

suffering from symphysis pubis diastasis (SPD) as this may aggravate the condition (Fig. 6.4B).

Why? These are techniques that Ikuyo Hosaka often used and are now used by her granddaughter Naoko. They can be useful for backache, especially that caused by the sacro-iliac joint. One of the two ways usually feels more comfortable for the mother, so work with this one. It also can help to focus the energy – either to the back or the front. The sacral opening can be useful for women with SPD as it draws energy to the front.

Specific sacral groove work

Although the general pressure can be very effective, sometimes it is not enough. This is when it is helpful to apply strong pressure into the sacral

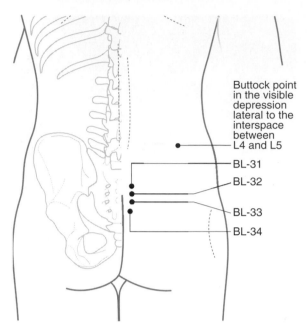

Buttock point in the visible depression lateral to the interspace between L4 and L5

BL-31

BL-32

BL-33

BL-34

Figure 6.5   Points BL31–34 and the buttock point.

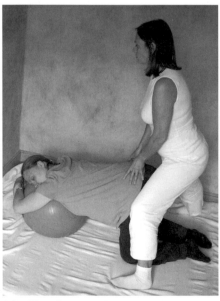

Figure 6.6   Thumb massaging to find the sacral points. Note the position of the practitioner and how the shoulders are relaxed and the movement comes from the hara.

grooves/foramen (Figs 6.5 and 6.6). The sacral grooves are four pairs of points on the sacrum – on some people they are easy to find, and on others not so. They are four holes in the bone of

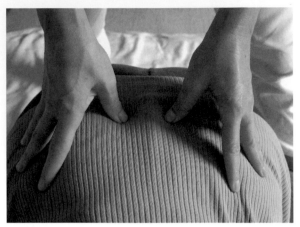

Figure 6.7   Thumb massaging to find the sacral points. Note how the rest of the hand acts as the mother hand.

the sacrum through which the sacral nerves pass – usually about a thumbwidth out from the midline, although it varies from person to person depending on the size of their bones. You can locate them by feeling from the top of the iliac crest (hip bone). Following its curve down, you will reach the top points. An alternative way of locating them is by feeling the tail bone and feeling up for the first set of points. Begin at the top or the bottom and place the pads of your thumbs in a pair of points (Fig. 6.7). Start gently massaging around the dip with small circling movements; this allows your thumbs to settle in the centre of the point. Then lean in with your bodyweight to apply static pressure. Make sure that the thumb joint is straight. The fingers of the rest of your hand act as the mother hand.

To increase the pressure in the points, you can work them one at a time. In this case, place one thumb on top of the other (Fig. 6.8). Lean in deeply. Make sure your fingers support your hand by making contact with the body. The fingers act as the mother hand.

You can also use your knuckles in these points, either one at a time or in pairs. To do this, bend your fingers into your palm. Place the second knuckle joint away from the fingertip of the index finger into one of the points. If you are working one point at a time, take your other hand and wrap it round the working hand so that it both gives stability to the working hand and is in contact with the mother's body – a double-acting

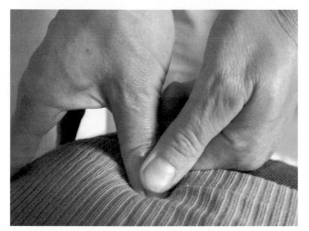

Figure 6.8 Using one thumb on top of the other.

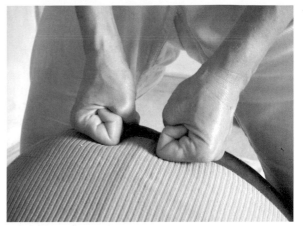

Figure 6.10 Using the rolling knuckle technique on the sacrum.

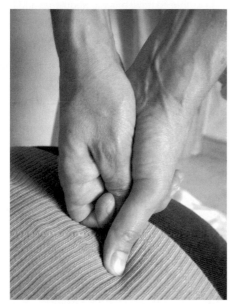

Figure 6.9 Using the knuckle in the point. Note the mother hand wrapped around to support the working hand, and the thumb and fingers acting as the mother hand.

mother hand (Fig. 6.9). If you are working both sides at the same time, place the knuckles of both index fingers in the highest sacral point and lean in with your body-weight (Fig. 6.10). You can then roll your knuckles in a straight line down the sacrum as far as they will go. You can repeat this, starting with your index finger knuckle in the second point down.

Work all pairs of points – you may well find that some points are easier to feel, some feel more tender to touch, and some you can go into quite deeply. This is your diagnosis of Kyo and Jitsu. Work first with the more Kyo. You may find the mother wants you to stay there. You may find one side is Kyo and the other side is Jitsu – work until you balance them out.

You can use the same techniques, but just working one side, with the mother in the side-lying position. Turn your hips and hara to face the mother's body and focus mostly on the grooves on the side uppermost, although sometimes it may be possible to work both sides.

After working, it is quite a good idea to do some of the hand-over-hand stroking over the buttocks and down the legs to allow the energy released to flow and be integrated by the rest of the body.

Why? This is another way of balancing the energy of the sacrum. The points are on the Bladder meridian. They are important points for genital disorders in men and women, and for prolapse of the uterus and sterility in women. All tonify the Kidneys and benefit Essence, and so tonify the whole body. They are also used to strengthen the lower back and knees. They can be used for difficult urination. They help to release energy through to the uterus – women often feel a comforting warmth in the uterus as these points are worked. They relate to the sacral nerves and thus will help with pain relief in labour. It is the sacral nerves that supply the lower segment of the uterus and the perineum and lower vagina. This means that in labour we tend to work down the points as labour progresses.

Tightness in these points, especially more on one side than the other, can often indicate the baby is stuck on the side where the energy is Jitsu. By releasing the Jitsu, the baby will often change position.

They are most commonly used during first-stage contractions for pain relief and to help the contractions to be more effective. Usually they are used during contractions – many women need only these for pain relief through the whole labour. It can be useful to teach them to the partner. You just need to work as long as the mother wants. Often, in between contractions, the mother appreciates the stroking techniques. They can be used in second stage if the contractions seem ineffective to focus the mother's energy, and in third stage for uterine bleeding.

BL-31 is in the top sacral groove. BL-32 is in the second sacral groove, counting downwards towards the coccyx. It is the most important as it tonifies the Kidneys and the Essence. It is used for infertility, prolapse of the anus and uterus, and stimulates ascending Ki. BL-33 has more of an effect on the Bladder and promotes, with BL-20, formation of Blood in Blood deficiency. BL-34 regulates Ki and Blood, and can be used for uterine bleeding, especially third-stage bleeding.

Buttock points

These two points are known as extra points – they are not on any particular meridian. One on each side, they are known as the lumbar eye – and are level with the fourth lumbar vertebrae, about 3.5 thumbwidths from the midline. They are often seen quite clearly as dimples in the buttock below the iliac crest.

To work, you place a thumb in the point on each side and use your fingers to cup round the top of the iliac crest (Fig. 6.11). The fingers act as the mother hand. Lean in at 90° with your thumbs while drawing back with your thumbs. You can also work one point at a time with one thumb on top of the other.

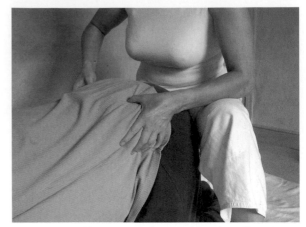

Figure 6.11 Working with the buttock points. Note the position of the practitioner with the hara behind the hands. Remember to have relaxed shoulders and lean from the hara.

Why? They are good points for strengthening the Kidneys and supporting the lumbar spine. They can be helpful for exhaustion, backache and pain relief. They can be used to help open up the pelvis during either first- or second-stage contractions. Ikuyo Hosaka in her practice in Japan often used them.

Drawing up GV energy or the hooking technique

This can be done if the mother is bearing down before the cervix is fully dilated and the baby's head can be felt pushing against the perineum. If the mother is on all fours, place one hand on the perineum. The palm should be over the top of the baby's head. Place the other hand on the sacrum with its fingers pointing down to the coccyx. Draw up strongly with the hand on the perineum and draw down with the hand on the sacrum (Fig. 6.12).

Why? This allows the Governing Vessel energy to flow down to the perineum and then strongly up again. This helps the baby to stay in the uterus until the cervix is fully dilated and takes away the mother's urge to bear down. This is another one of Ikuyo's techniques which Naoko taught me. Naoko has used it often in her practice and so now have many other midwives who have done my course.

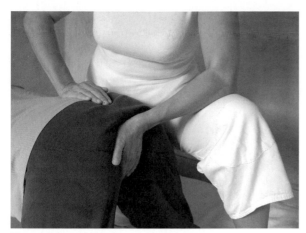

Figure 6.12 Drawing up the GV energy or hooking technique. Note the position of the hands and the practitioner's body.

Case study 6.1   Hooking case study – an independent midwife

A primigravida woman started to have mild contractions every 7 min a few hours after she had had a show. Six hours on her contractions were regular at 5 min and slightly stronger. At this stage the SP-6 tsubo was worked on both legs alternately. The contractions were much stronger 20 min later.

Within 3 h the contractions were strong and regular every 2–3 min. By this time she was having more of a lower back pain, especially with contractions. Pressure was applied using both hands on the B-27 to B-34 tsubo area, but when she had a contraction, each tsubo was worked on with both thumbs in the direction of the coccyx to relieve the pain.

Two hours on she felt rectal pressure with each contraction. The cervix was 8–9 cm and the head was high. In order for her not to bear down when having contractions, one hand was left on her sacral area and the other hand was placed along the coccyx to the perineum, hooking the fingers around. With the contractions, the hand on the sacrum applied firm pressure to the area, and the hooking hand put pressure on to the curvature of the area, relieving the rectal pressure. This was continued until the hooking hand could feel the head descending on to the fingers. This ensured that the head was low. The woman also felt a strong urge to push and I could see her body voluntarily pushing. With six pushes she gave birth to a female infant.

Box 6.2   Bladder partner exercise – sitting back to back

This is the exercise we did in the basic principles section on pages 75–76. It is a good exercise to help make people aware of the energy of the back as well as to show them how shiatsu works; it can be included in antenatal classes to encourage mothers and partners to work together.

Neck, head and shoulder routines

The neck and head are important to work because tension is often stored here. In labour, many women clench their jaws and tighten their shoulders. This can give rise, not only to generalized tightness in the neck and shoulders, but also to specific symptoms such as headaches, nasal congestion and emotional tension.

Neck work can be useful at all stages of labour. It can help with pain relief. Allowing energy to flow will also help the body to do whatever it needs to. It is especially important to support wood energy in the second stage. If you notice a big difference in tightness, i.e. Jitsu, between the two sides, or if it is very Jitsu, this can be an indication of the baby being stuck. As with this kind of tightness in the sacrum, by balancing the Kyo and Jitsu, it is often possible to change the baby's position during labour.

There is a relationship between the neck and the sacrum, both structurally and energetically. The sacral points are on the Bladder and so are the points on the back of the neck each side of the vertebrae. The Bladder begins at the inner corner of the eye and goes over the head to the neck. If the mother is experiencing pain in the sacrum and working directly on the points there seems too intense or uncomfortable, then working in the neck is a good alternative.

The shoulders are closely linked in with the head. Often tension from the head will manifest in the shoulders and vice versa. The side of the neck, top of the shoulder and around the shoulder blade relate to the Gall Bladder meridian – this is wood energy. There is a tendency for it to be Jitsu as out-of-balance wood energy often rises and gets stuck here. This is aggravated by the sedentary lifestyle of modern culture – especially sitting at a desk or driving. In labour, if women are leaning forward or using the all fours position, they may hold tension here.

In shiatsu, we consider that the shoulders are related to the hips – if the shoulders are tight, then so are the hips. The hips also relate to wood energy – the Gall Bladder meridian is the main meridian which passes through here. If the hips are too tight, or too loose, energy may not flow well in second stage and the birth may be more difficult.

There is a close link between water and wood. In labour, the first stage is water energy and the second stage is wood. Wood is related to strong physical downward movement and the delivery of the baby. From their element relationship, we say that water needs to moisten the wood – like watering a tree or plants. Water is essential for life and growth. If there is not much water, the tree will dry, and wither and die. It will become gnarled and tight. We can say that tightness in the neck and shoulders is a sign that water energy may not be flowing. By working water, wood can soften.

The throat is considered to be related to the cervix and the perineum. This is largely through the link with the whole digestive tract, which is seen as beginning with the mouth and ending with the anus and urethra. This is, in a large part, Governing Vessel and Conception Vessel energy. The starting and ending points of these meridians are on the perineum and around the mouth. It also links with metal energy – Lung and Large Intestine – the taking in of nutrients in the form of air and letting go at the other end in the form of body wastes.

Box 6.3   Wood energy visualization – the tree

Sit and begin to breathe into your hara.

As you relax, begin to feel that your legs are like roots going down into the earth. Feel them burrowing through the earth and pushing further and further downwards. Feel the darkness and warmth and resistance of the earth. Feel the roots reaching right into the centre of the earth.

Stay with this connection for a while.

Now begin to feel that there is also a flow of energy moving up your body from your hara. Feel that your body is like the trunk of a tree, very solid and firm, connected downwards through the roots but with an energy spreading into the arms. Allow yourself to feel the strength and flexibility of the trunk. Feel the support.

After a while, feel energy rising out of the trunk into your arms and head. This is the energy of the branches and the leaves. Feel branches moving out and up. Feel the leaves uncurling. Feel movement in the leaves and branches, movement and lightness. Feel the air and space around you.

In labour, if you feel there is tightness in the upper body connect with the movement of the leaves. If you feel there is no energy moving down into the perineum, connect with the energy of the roots. If you feel indecisive, unclear, unfocused, focus on the energy of the trunk.

Box 6.4   Wood exercise – circling together

Sit on the floor facing your partner, have your legs apart. Try to keep your legs as straight as you comfortably can and place the soles of your feet against your partner's soles. Hold out your arms and hold each other's wrists. Spend some time breathing deeply and being aware of your partner's breathing. Then begin to do some circling movements, moving from your hips. Keep your legs, back and arms as straight as you can. Circle slowly to start with in one direction. Find a rhythm to the movement. Now reverse the direction of the movement. After a while slow the movement down and rest. Then one of you leans forwards, keeping their legs as straight as they comfortably can and so the other will lean back. Stay for a few breaths and relax. If the person leaning forward wants to go further then they can do so, but it is important that the person leaning back doesn't pull or force their partner to lean forwards. Then come to the centre and the other person goes back and their partner goes forward.

Do not do this exercise if you have pain in the pubic bone.

Box 6.5   Exercise for the jaw and cervix

Clench your jaw and grit your teeth. Observe what happens to your breathing and also what you can feel in your perineum and vaginal area. Now open the jaw and make an aah sound. Now observe your breathing and your perineum.

What did you find? You should notice that as you relax your jaw and make an aah sound, you breathe out more deeply, and the perineum and vagina relax.

Basic techniques

The amount of pressure you use on the neck is going to be much less than you used on the sacrum. You can work close to the vertebrae but you need to check that there is no discomfort. People tend to love or hate their neck being worked – it is a more sensitive area than the lower back, so do get feedback about what feels good. Some people really do not like their necks being worked – you need to respect this.

Your body position for most of these techniques is facing the base of the neck. Make sure that you are comfortable.

Neck holds

Begin by generally relaxing the neck through cupping the base of the occiput with the 'web' of one hand, i.e. the area between your thumb and index finger. Place the other hand over the mother's forehead, being careful not to cover her eyes (Fig. 6.13). Gently use the mother hand (the hand on the forehead) to ease the head back on to the working hand. This gives a generalized pressure on the base of the skull.

Stroking

You may want to use light hand-over-hand stroking over the head and down the shoulders to move energy and relax.

Remember, slower stroking is more tonifying – to draw energy in. Faster strokes are more sedating – to take energy away.

Usually, there tends to be too much energy in the head, so you will find you tend to want to stroke down over the top of the head and over the shoulders.

Palm holds

Place the palm of one hand to cup over a Kyo point and the palm of the other hand to cup over a Jitsu point. Hold the two and focus on the energy shifting between the two.

Why?   All of these are for relaxing the neck and freeing energy.

More complex techniques

Meridian pathways

There are some specific meridians and points that are useful in the neck (Fig. 6.14). If you identify these pathways, then you can focus your palming or stroking along the one you feel most relevant.

All the following points are worked in a similar way, although the angle of pressure may change depending on where the point lies. Hold your thumb in the point, with your fingers of this hand resting where they are comfortable on the head. Place your mother hand on the forehead. Use your mother hand to guide the head into the working thumb or simply to provide some balancing pressure – remembering the principle of equal pressure between the two hands. Do this slowly, building up to maximum pressure. Repeat a few times and then repeat on the other side.

Bladder 10 (BL-10)   To locate this, place your thumbs each side of the cervical vertebrae about 1.5 thumbwidths from the centre. Slide up to the base of the skull – you will find a hollow. It is on the side of the trapezius muscle about half an inch above the hairline in the slight depression about an inch to each side of the spinal groove.

Since the point lies under the occiput, then instead of a 90° angle, you need to angle so as to

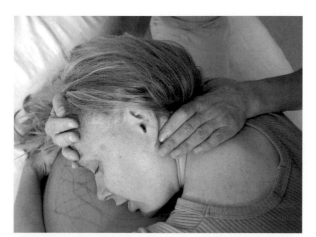

Figure 6.13   Neck hold. Note the mother hand on the forehead and the working hand on the base of the skull. The practitioner needs to remember to have the hara close to the head and their own shoulders relaxed.

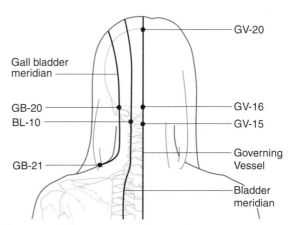

Figure 6.14   Points and meridian pathways of the neck. The pathways of the Bladder meridian, the Gall Bladder, Governing Vessel and the locations of the points BL-10, GV-15, GV-16, GV-20, GB-20 and GB-21.

'hook' under the bone (Fig. 6.15). Apply the pressure towards the mother hand to establish the two-hand connection.

Why?   It is known as the 'celestial pillar'. It clears the head, and is a useful point for occipital or vertical headaches. It can ease stiff necks and headaches. Because of its close relationship to the brain, it clears the brain, stimulates memory and concentration. It has a special effect on the eyes, helping to increase vision, and can clear nasal congestion. It can help with backache and wobbly legs which seem unable to support the body. It helps with water energy flow and therefore can be very calming and relaxing.

Governing Vessel 15 and 16 (GV-15/16) GV-16 is on the midline of the nape of the neck in the depression just below the external occipital protruberance (i.e. the bony prominence in the base of the skull). GV-15 is 0.5 thumbwidth below it – often between BL-10.

Work in the same way as BL-10, except angle your pressure directly in a 90° angle. You will find that you can't apply as much pressure as with BL-10.

Why?   Both these points affect Governing Vessel energy and benefit the neck and spine. They can gather the energy of the body at times of change or when the energy is stuck.

GV-15 clears the mind, stimulates speech and is indicated for heaviness of the head or loss of consciousness. GV-16 is said to nourish the brain and clear headaches.

Gall Bladder 20 (GB-20)   This is an inch above the hairline in the depression between the sterno-cleido-mastoid and the upper portion of the trapezius muscles. Locate BL-10, then slide up and slightly out until you come to a protrusion of the skull. The point lies just below and to the outside.

Work in the same way as BL-10, except that you need to angle the pressure in at 45°, i.e diagonally, while also 'hooking' under the bone.

Why?   This releases tension in the head, especially relating to headaches in the side of the head. It helps release tightness in the wood energy.

Five-point head hold technique   If you are able to, stand in front of the mother so that her face is in front of you and you can place your fingers under her occiput, so that when you lean, her head and spine may extend. If you have to stand behind her, you will have to hold as many of the points as best you can.

Place your index fingers one on top of each other into GV-15, then place your middle fingers each side in BL-10, then your ring fingers in GB-20. Hook the fingers under the points and bring your palms onto the skull so that they are cupping it. Bring your thumbs one on top of each other onto the skull wherever they land. Your palms are the mother hand so you need a good connection with them. Gently lean your hara back and draw your hands towards you. This way you stimulate all five points at the same time (Fig. 6.16). Notice which are the most Kyo and

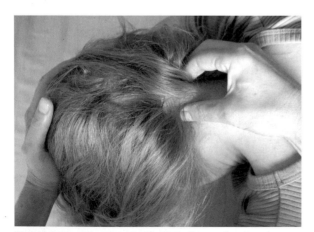

Figure 6.15   Working BL-10. Note the mother hand on the forehead.

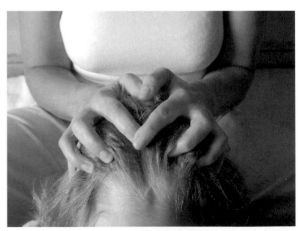

Figure 6.16   Five-point hold technique.

Jitsu – hold the Kyo and use more dispersing techniques for the Jitsu. To disperse while you are holding, you can go in a little quicker and sharper; you can also use gentle vibration movements with the thumbs/fingers.

Why?   This was used traditionally by midwives in Japan and is still used today. It is a technique passed down from Ikuyo via Naoko. It frees the energy of all the important points at the base of the occiput. It can sometimes be more effective to work them all together.

Governing Vessel 20 (GV-20)   This is right at the top of the head. To find it, place the heels of your hands on the anterior and posterior hairlines and extend the middle fingers towards each other. It is 1 thumbwidth anterior to where the middle fingers meet. You can also extend a line from the tip of each ear to the top of the head. The point is usually just in front of the crown of the head.

Place one thumb on top of the other on the point, and cup the head with the rest of your hand and fingers. The thumbs are the 'working hand' and the rest of the hand the 'mother hand' (Fig. 6.17). You can either focus on gentle pressure down the body, along the spine. Or you can focus on drawing the energy up – depending on what you need to do.

Why?   It is the meeting point of all the Yang channels which carry Yang to the head, and therefore has the effect of clearing the mind and lifting the spirits. It also strengthens the ascending function

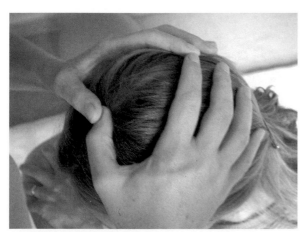

Figure 6.17   Working GV-20.

of the Spleen and is used for prolapse of internal organs such as the stomach, uterus, bladder, anus or vagina; it can also be used to revive an unconscious person. It has a powerful effect on either raising or lowering blood pressure, depending on whether your intention in using it is to send energy down the body, or draw energy up the body. At any time in labour, if the mother is exhausted or running out of energy, especially if you feel that she is 'blanking out', it can help draw her energy up. It can also be a point to promote relaxation at any stage of labour. You can focus with upward intention to help draw Yang energy up if the mother wants to bear down before she is ready, and it works well in conjunction with the GV drawing-up hold on pages 96–97. You can focus with downward intention to promote movement of Yang energy downwards in transition or during second or third stage.

Shoulder leaning

A good way of working the shoulders is with your forearms. This also provides an opportunity to rest your hands. You can either stand behind the mother or stand face to face, depending on her position, so that you can place your forearms over the top of the shoulders and lean in the direction of her spine down towards her feet (Fig. 6.18). You can do some stroking and rolling with forearms. This helps release the Jitsu.

Shoulder point not for use in pregnancy

Gall Bladder 21 (GB-21)   This is in the hollow on top of the shoulder, straight up from the nipple when you are standing. It is in the highest point of the muscle on the shoulder. An accurate way is to measure from the seventh cervical vertebrae (GV-14) out along the neck. It is midway between here and the tip of the acromium process of the scapula (Fig. 6.19), at the crest of the trapezius muscle.

This can be incorporated in a shoulder massage which is relaxing for the woman in labour. You can place your thumbs directly in the points and lean down in the same way as for general shoulder relaxing.

Why?   It is an extremely powerful point as it shifts energy quite dramatically. It is one of the

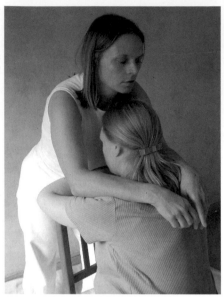

Figure 6.18 Leaning with forearms onto the shoulders. Note the position of the practitioner's body, the hara facing the head and shoulders relaxed.

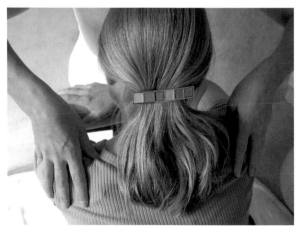

Figure 6.19 Working GB-21.

points that should not be stimulated in pregnancy, except for induction, as it moves energy downward very strongly and can stimulate contractions. It therefore can be used for induction or at any stage of labour to stimulate downward movement of the baby or contractions. It can be used in third stage for helping to deliver retained placentas. It relaxes tension in the shoulder, neck and jaw. Some women enjoy this point for pain relief for hours in labour. It can also help with poor lactation.

Case study 6.2   Retained placenta, by a senior midwife

K was 41 weeks pregnant with her first baby. She had no past medical or gynaecological history and had practised yoga throughout her pregnancy. She had been considering acupuncture if she needed an induction of labour. She was admitted in strong labour, deemed to be in transition.

The first stage was spent at home and lasted only 4 h. She delivered within half an hour of admission. She opted for physiological management of the third stage and was waiting as she was not bleeding. One hour after the birth there was no sign that the placenta was going to be delivered. I attended then. After explaining to K about shiatsu, which she knew about, I proceeded to make contact with her body by moving the Ki from the Jitsu area which was in the heart region to the uterus which I felt was Kyo. I did this by palming with my left hand from the heart to the uterus. My right hand, the mother hand, was stationary on the uterus. My next approach was applying acupressure to the GB-21 point and LI-4. Almost immediately, she felt some strong contractions and the placenta and membranes were delivered complete by maternal effort 5 min later. K and her partner were very pleased with the outcome. The prospect of having a spinal anaesthetic for manual removal was avoided.

Personal reflection
A very satisfying outcome. K said that she would have been very disappointed if she had to be transferred to the operating theatre for a manual removal of the placenta under anaesthetic.

Case study 6.3   Labour shiatsu – home birth for a first baby – a community midwife

On arrival at P's flat, I found her in the bedroom, tensing up with the contractions and not coping very well. Her husband was trying to comfort her through his own obvious distress. I went directly over to her, dropping my bag at the door and proceeded to lay my hands on her shoulders (Gall Bladder 21). I verbally reassured her, calming her and encouraging her into a slow breathing rhythm. When the next contraction came and P looked as though she was becoming distressed, I gently leaned into the sacral points with my thumbs, breathing with P until the contraction had passed. As I listened to the information about the labour, I provided physical and emotional support, holding the sides of P's head, gently continuing the breathing in union with hers. The points at the back of the head, GB-20, BL-10 and GV-15, were soothing and energy giving as I gently worked over them.

I was thus able to get P to relax enough for examination and give myself a good idea of the strength and frequency of the contractions. As expected, P was in established labour and the cervix, effaced, was 4–5 cm dilated. My presence calmed her enough for her to draw on her own resources and she was coping beautifully with the contractions. I felt that an hour in the bath would assist dilatation at this point and she was keen to try this. Her husband and I assisted her into the bath. I guided her through a couple of contractions and saw her melt in an endorphic state.

P was 8 cm dilated after the bath and a second midwife was found to bring the resuscitation equipment and provide support if needed for the birth.

P had tiny hips! The second stage of baby's descent to birth was thus assisted by innovative positions and many changes of these. I had to keep an eye on the baby's progress so I asked her partner to sit behind her on the toilet seat, supporting her for contractions and holding GB-21 to encourage descent. At 05.10 a healthy baby boy was born, screaming for a full 20 min. P was not even grazed by the birth.

I visited P postnatally and we were both delighted and grateful for the shiatsu, which made all the difference to this experience and was a very valuable and supportive tool for me as a midwife.

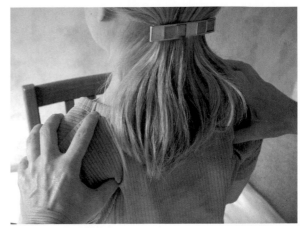

Figure 6.20   Working the three-point shoulder hold.

Case study 6.4   Induction of labour – midwife and partner working together – a hospital midwife

S was a 39-year-old gravida 4, para 3. She had an induction for both her first and second pregnancies. I saw her when she was 7 days post-dates and showed her some hara breathing, all fours and squatting positions, and taught her how to use GB-21. I spent probably about 10–15 min with her and then she went home. S told me that her husband had used GB-21 twice for 10 min each time. He then felt completely drained and went to sleep for one and half hours. Just after this time S started to have contractions. She went on to have a 4-h 20-min labour and gave birth to a baby boy of 4040 g, apgar 9 and 10. The placenta was delivered 15 min later – it was large and had an irregular edge with a retro-placental clot. The perineum was intact and blood loss was 500 ml. S was very pleased with the effect of her shiatsu.

Shoulder opening – three-point hold (from Ikuyo Hosaka)

Standing behind the mother, place your hands on the top of her shoulders. Place your index finger on the top around GB-21, your thumb round the back on the shoulder blade and your other fingers around the front where they feel comfortable (Fig. 6.20). As the mother breathes out, lean down with the index finger in GB-21 and ease the shoulder back onto the thumb.

Why?   This is another traditional technique from Ikuyo. It is very powerful for releasing the shoulder and freeing wood energy.

Abdominal work

The abdomen is the energy of the hara. The hara in fact covers a larger area than what we consider to be the abdomen – its lower border is the pubic bone, its side borders are just along the anterior iliac spines and the upper border is under the ribs. You may be familiar with important energy centres in the hara such as Dantian – Conception Vessel 4 (CV-4). This point, 3 thumbwidths below the navel on the midline, is given great importance in most Eastern martial art and bodywork traditions.

In shiatsu, Masunaga (1977) developed the use of diagnostic areas for the 12 main meridians. There are in fact many traditions of using the hara for diagnosis of all energies in the body. In traditional acupuncture, like there are organ points along the Bladder meridian, there are also many important organ points on the Conception Vessel which runs along the midline of the body. Other important meridians which pass through the hara are: the Penetrating Vessel and Kidney meridians (which share the same pathways), the Stomach meridian, Girdle Vessel, Heart–Uterus and Kidney–Uterus.

The lower hara is considered to be especially important. It represents the deepest energy of the body related to original Ki and Essence. GV-4 on the back between the second and third lumbar vertebrae, the Ming Men, is considered to be the source of all energy in the body and its action is said to move towards the front and affect the energy of the hara.

Work on the hara strongly and directly affects all the abdominal organs, including the uterus. In pregnancy, this includes the fetus and the placenta. The hara helps the mother make emotional connections with her baby – prenatal bonding; it also helps to calm the baby and is useful in cases of fetal distress in labour.

As the hara is the physical centre of the body and the centre is said to represent earth energy, we can say that it is linked with earth energy as well as with that of the extraordinary vessels. Without earth, there is no place for the other energies to be grounded. Earth provides the link between our Essence, our constitutional energy, and our Ki, our day-to-day energy, through the link with food Ki.

The Yin meridians of Spleen, Liver and Kidney all pass through and dominate the energy of the lower abdomen. These are all important in labour.

It is therefore of vital importance to ensure the smooth flow of energy through the hara. This can tend to get blocked in pregnancy as the baby physically grows bigger. Breathing will help with this energy flow, as will gentle holding techniques. There are some simple techniques that are useful to show to the parents as they provide a way of linking them directly with their baby.

Box 6.6   Earth visualization

This can be done either sitting, squatting or in all fours. It is useful to do this in pregnancy, especially in the first trimester, as the energy of the baby is settling in the uterus.

Breathe deeply into your hara and relax with each out-breath.

As you breathe out, begin to focus on the point CV-4, Dantian, 3 thumbwidths below the navel. First of all be aware of the surface of the point, the skin and the flesh, and the movement in with the out-breath and out with the in-breath.

After a while, gradually begin to allow your attention to go deeper inside your body to the centre. Be aware of the colours and sensations you feel as you do this.

After a while, imagine that you are surrounded by earth in a way that feels supportive. It is nourishing you. You are like a seed in the earth, able to grow and develop. Be aware of the browns and oranges of the earth.

Be aware of your navel and feel the umbilical cord connecting you with your mother.

Be aware of the energetic connection of earth mothering energy (rather than your physical mother).

After a while ease out of these connections and be aware of your body as it is now and its connection with the ground where you are in this moment.

When you are ready, open your eyes.

Box 6.7   Earth exercise – the squat with partner

Most women need to practise the squat, as although it is instinctive, most of us have forgotten how to use our bodies in this way. It is best to begin in the second trimester when the pregnancy is established and should not be done if there is any bleeding. It is not advisable to do this if the baby is breech or if you have symphysis pubis diastasis. Do not stay in the position if you have varicose veins. There is debate over deep squatting in the last trimester (Sutton & Scott 1996) but if the baby is anterior cephalic and the mother is comfortable, I find that it is fine to continue. If the baby is transverse or oblique it is usually uncomfortable. If the baby is posterior, small amounts of squatting combined with more emphasis on all fours is fine. The benefits of the squat, on opening the hips and strengthening the pelvic floor and muscles of the legs and back, make it worth continuing if in smaller amounts. The main guidance for any of the exercises for mother or midwife is if it is uncomfortable in any way, do not continue.

Stand and face a partner with your arms outstretched. Have your feet a little wider than hip width apart, although at any point of the exercise, change your foot position if it feels uncomfortable. Hold each other's hands at the wrists. Make sure that you are standing upright and not leaning backwards. Close your eyes and be aware of each other's breathing. After a while open your eyes and begin to do some swaying movements from side to side. When you feel confident with these, do some circling movements. Be aware of how you support each other's weight. When you are ready, come back to resting once more.

Then as you both breathe out, sink down into the full squatting position (Fig. 6.21). You should find this much easier to do than squatting on your own. Make sure that your arms are fully extended. Position your feet so that your weight is in the centre of the foot and you are not putting strain on your ankles. Stay in this position as long as you feel comfortable. As you stay in this position feel the connection of your feet with the floor. Be aware of the earth beneath you.

When you are ready, as you both breathe out, come back to standing once more.

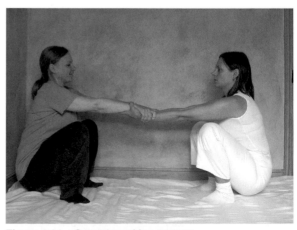

Figure 6.21   Squatting with a partner.

Basic techniques

General abdominal pressures

You can do this with the mother in a variety of different positions. The most helpful position for labour is in all fours. She could also be in the left lateral position or even standing. You need to make sure that you are in a position where you are comfortable and your hara is close to the mother (Fig. 6.22).

Begin by placing one hand on the mother's abdomen and one hand on her lower back; how high up or low down you have this depends on the most comfortable place for the mother. Having the hand on the lower back tends to allow the mother to feel less invaded, more supported and to experience a connection which is deep inside her body from front to back. Just allow your hands to mould to the shape of the mother's body and to rest there for a while. Feel the connection between your two hands and feel the movement of the mother's breathing, drawing your hands gently together as she breathes out and gently pushing them away as she breathes in. This is very much like the hara breathing exercise (page 75) – but doing it with someone else. After a while, begin to apply gentle pressure as the mother breathes out, by drawing your two hands together. As the mother breathes in, feel your hands being pushed

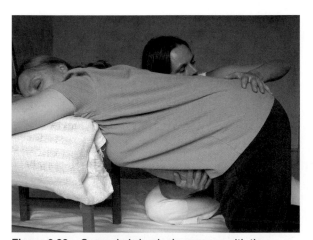

Figure 6.22   General abdominal pressure, with the mother hand on the back and the working hand on the abdomen. Note that the working hand needs to move up to the mother hand and the angle of pressure into the body needs to be at 90°. The practitioner needs to have their shoulders relaxed and their hara close to the mother's body.

away and release the pressure, but keep the contact. Be aware of the baby in the womb. Connect with how much pressure feels appropriate. Make sure that the pressure is going in at 90° to the mother's body – your hand should not feel like it is dragging up or down on the abdomen, simply going inwards.

You can work different places on the front by moving the hand. Begin by sliding the hand round, as though you're moving one or two hours in a clockwise direction round the abdomen. On the new place, repeat the pressure. Remember that the amount of pressure will vary from place to place. You may also find that some places really draw you in and you want to stay for longer – these are the Kyo areas. Other places may feel firmer and push you away so that you may only want to stay for a few out-breaths. These are the Jitsu areas. It is important to work in a clockwise direction to follow the movement of the intestines. Keep the hand on the sacrum/lower back stable; this is the mother hand.

You can also intersperse some clockwise stroking movements on the abdomen with these pressures. This is more dispersing, although you can do it slowly with the focus of calming, in which case it is more tonifiying.

Why?   It helps the mother to connect with her breathing and to breathe deeper. It helps to bring the focus on to the baby as opposed to the pain. It can help to calm the baby.

Obviously, there may well be times in labour when the mother doesn't want any contact with her abdomen, and for some women this could be throughout labour. However, some women do appreciate the holding on the abdomen. This is a simple useful exercise to show partners and helps both mother and father connect more with their baby. In this case, you can get the partner to focus not only on Kyo and Jitsu – in an antenatal class I wouldn't mention these terms – but also to be aware of the baby's body and how the baby is responding to the touch.

Kidney–Uterus

Similar to the above, but this time, place your hand on the back over one of the mother's kidneys. Visualize energy from the kidney moving through into the hara. Feel a strong connection with this hand. You can move the hand over the abdomen as before, connecting with the uterus and the baby. You can then move on to placing your mother hand over the other kidney and repeating.

Why?   It gives a more specific focus to the hara work – focusing on the Kidney which relates to sending Essence to the Uterus. It can be especially helpful at times when the mother is completely exhausted, or when the contractions seem to be ineffective, at any stage of labour. It is also a very useful technique for calming a distressed baby.

Girdle Vessel

Stand behind the mother, with your hara close against her back. Your hara is going to act like the mother hand. Place your two hands one on top of the other over the abdomen, with the little finger sides over the top edge of the pubic bone and your palms cupping over the lower hara (Fig. 6.23A). You can check where it feels most comfortable. Stay for a little while, applying gentle pressures as in the general abdominal work, remembering to have the pressure going at 90° directly into the mother's body, which is going to be drawing your hands inwards to your hara. After a while, as the mother breathes out, gently draw your hands in a firm stroking movement, from the front to the back of her body, passing around her hips and ending up at about the level of the second to third

lumbar vertebra (Fig. 6.23B and C). Focus your attention on the inside of her body as well as the outside, so that a deep connection is made. Rest your hands on her back to finish.

From the finishing position, do the reverse. Slide your hands from back to front.

Some mothers are clear that they prefer the movement in one way only, others like both directions. If you are able to get a sense of whether it is the back or the hara that feels more Kyo or Jitsu, then you will find that you need to move from the Jitsu to the Kyo.

For women with symphysis pubis diastasis, it is usually best to draw the energy to the pubis as there is often a lack of energy here. However, as this is not a strong opening technique (like the sacral opening), then it can also be used the other way if there is too much energy in the front.

Why?   As the Girdle Vessel is about linking from front to back, it can help to balance the two. It can be useful if the mother has strong backache where you feel she is holding on to tension and the energy is low in the uterus, so that it is not dilating. This is often the pattern if the baby is stuck, in either first or second stage, in an awkward position, e.g. posterior or asynclitic. By moving the energy from front to back, you can free the baby to move. The Girdle Vessel is closely related to wood energy (via its connections with

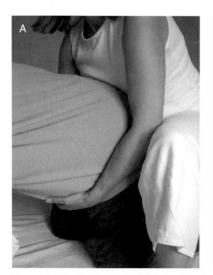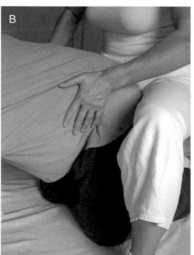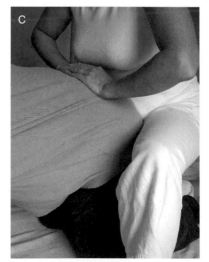

Figure 6.23   A, B, C: Stroking the Girdle Vessel meridian. Note the partner's hara, which is close to the mother's back, even leaning onto her back. The shoulders need to be relaxed.

the Liver and Gall Bladder meridians) which needs to flow in second stage and so can help with uncoordinated contractions in either first or second stage or at any time when you feel energy is blocked in some way in the pelvis. Linked with the Spleen, Liver and Kidney energies, it is a good linking meridian to support the deep abdominal muscles and uterine ligaments. It can be useful for supporting a mother who has a weak symphysis pubis or sacro-iliac joint. It can also help focus second-stage contractions. It can be very calming for mother and baby as it is working to balance deep energies in the body.

Connecting CV and GV through their lower pathways

This is easiest to do in a position where you can reach both the front and back of the mother – such as all fours, standing, side lying. Place either the little finger side of one hand, or your middle finger tip on CV-2, which is in the centre of the pubic bone along the top border. Place the middle finger tip of your other hand over GV-2, which is at the top of the coccyx where it joins the sacrum (Fig. 6.24). Let the palm of this hand act as the mother hand on the sacrum. Get a sense of which tsubo feels more Kyo and which more Jitsu.

Then focus your attention on the connection between the two which passes through the anus, through the centre of the perineum and up to the pubic bone. Imagine a pathway of energy flowing along this line from the Jitsu point to the Kyo point. Stay holding in this way until you feel warmth spreading along the line, or you feel the Kyo and the Jitsu evening out.

Why? This connects the lower pathways of the Governing Vessel and Conception Vessel and thus the perineum. Mothers often find that direct touch on the perineum in labour can feel invasive. For mothers who may have experienced sexual abuse, it may even be traumatic and this may be a reason why energy is not flowing here. Many women are disconnected from their perineums. This technique offers a safe, gentle way of getting energy to flow along here and can be especially useful in second stage for helping the mother to focus her energy onto the perineum.

More complex techniques

There are various points in the hara which can be worked. The mother can be in any position. Place your mother hand either on her lower back or on her abdomen, whichever is more comfortable. To make a more general connection with the points, you can use the palm of the working hand. To make a more specific connection use the thumb pad of the working hand (Fig. 6.25). If you apply

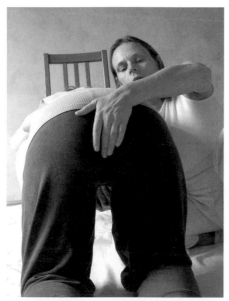

Figure 6.24 Connecting the Conception and Governing Vessels through their lower pathways. The focus needs to be on feeling the connection between the two hands.

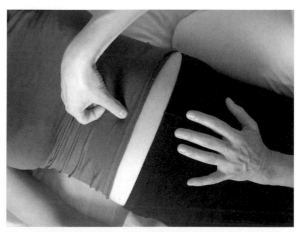

Figure 6.25 Using thumb pressures to work the upper part of the Conception Vessel. Note the mother hand on the lower hara and the working thumb which is supported by the rest of the hand.

all the basic principles, this work can be very powerful and feel relaxing. It is extremely important, more than anywhere else in the body, to work with the mother's out-breath and to increase the pressure gradually. The pressure can be very light so that you make more of an energetic connection. It may, however, feel appropriate to go in deeply – but of course you need to do this gradually, getting very good feedback from the mother. Often, people are quite scared of working on the abdomen, but it is safe if done properly. If you have any doubts, of course it is best to work too lightly than too deeply but you may be surprised how deep is comfortable. Think of how deeply you go in when you are palpating the baby – and sometimes this isn't all that comfortable for the mother.

Place either the palm or the thumb pad of your working hand on the relevant point and rest the fingers on the abdomen as support. As the mother breathes out, gradually increase thumb/palm pressure as much as is comfortable (remembering to increase pressure with the mother hand while you do this) and hold it until she breathes in again. Allow the movement of her abdomen to gradually push away the thumb as she breathes out, but remain in contact. Get a sense if the point is Kyo or Jitsu. If it is Kyo, then repeat this until you feel more energy coming into the point. If it is Jitsu, you could include a small circling or vibration movement as you work with the pressure.

The other way of working these points is to have two thumbs one on top of each other, and spread the rest of the hands on the abdomen to give support as mother hands. Work in the same way as before.

Use whichever way feels most comfortable for the mother.

Why? All the points are on the lower part of the Conception Vessel and relate closely to original Ki, Essence, the Uterus, Spleen, Liver and Kidney energy. They are good for exhaustion and depletion of these energies, and for helping energy to flow in the lower abdomen, including the lower burner; they can thus be useful at all stages of labour. They can all regulate uterine bleeding, ease pain in the uterus and lower abdomen, aid conception, expel a retained placenta and ease swelling of the cervix. They support bladder function, particularly retention of urine.

The points CV-3, CV-4 and CV-5

CV-3 is 4 thumbwidths below the navel on the midline (Fig. 6.26). It is an important point for regulating the Bladder. CV-4 is 3 thumbwidths below the navel on the midline (Fig. 6.26). Some traditions consider this to be one of the most important points in the body; one of its names is also Ming Men, indicating its close relationship with GV-4. It is especially powerful for benefiting the Essence and promoting fertility, and is said to be particularly calming when there is deep fear.

CV-5 is 2 thumbwidths below the navel on the midline (Fig. 6.26). This tends to be more important for regulating heat, as it is an important point for regulating the three burners/Triple Heater.

Any point along the midline of the front of the body can be worked as illustrated.

Other points (Fig. 6.26)

Zigong (Uterus point) is 3 thumbwidths lateral to CV-3. This promotes fertility, regulates Ki and stops pain; it is used for infertility and prolapse of the uterus.

Baomen (door of uterus) and Zihu (door of baby) are both 2 thumbwidths lateral to CV-4. Baomen is on the left and Zihu on the right. They are used for infertility, threatened miscarriage, retained placenta, difficult childbirth.

Legs and feet

The energy of the 12 meridians extends into the arms and legs. The Eastern view of the body is that the further points are away from the centre, the deeper their effect on the organs. Most acupuncturists tend to insert far more points around the wrists or feet. This fits in with the traditions of reflexology which consider that the whole body's energy is reflected in the feet. Many of the points for induction are around the feet, reflecting this deep internal connection. There is a grounding connection which is to do with earth and wood energy, and working with the feet can be a useful way of drawing energy down in labour. If there is too much energy in the neck and shoulders (Jitsu), you need to work the most Kyo

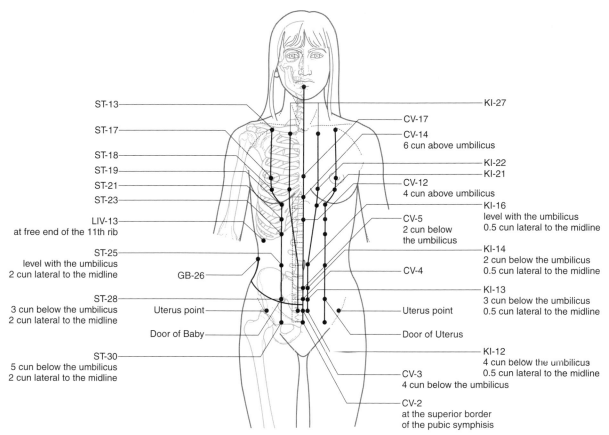

Figure 6.26 The hara – the main meridians, Conception Vessel (CV), Penetrating Vessel (PV) and Kidney (KI) and the main points, CV-3, CV-4, CV-5, Uterus point (three thumbwidths lateral to CV-3), door of the uterus and door of the baby (two thumbwidths lateral to CV-4) and ST-30.

part of the body, which is often the legs, to draw this energy down. Legs may get wobbly or shivery in labour, indicating that this basic body support system is having to do a lot of work to keep the body going.

Box 6.8 Exercise

Clench your toes. Feel what happens to your breathing and also to your pelvis.

Allow the toes to relax and feel the difference.

In Japan, in the last few weeks of pregnancy, women walk around with a little gadget between their toes to allow the energy to open up and flow. It is rather like what we use to open the toes to put on nail varnish. Another alternative is to put your fingers between your toes and wiggle them around. For a heavily pregnant mother this is quite difficult to do herself, so her partner could be involved. If the partner wants to get really intimate, they can suck the mother's toes.

Basic techniques

Meridian stroking technique

The mother can be standing or kneeling, leaning over the back of a chair. Start with one hand at the top of the outside leg and one hand at the inside of the ankle (Fig. 6.27).

Vigorously stroke the hand at the top down the outside of the leg, while at the same time moving the hand at the ankle up the inside of the leg.

Keep the movement flowing while you lightly move the hand which is now at the bottom, and the hand which is now at the top, back to where they started.

This technique can be done quite vigorously, provided there are no areas of varicose veins. It is an invigorating technique, good for stimulating circulation in the legs, as well as working on

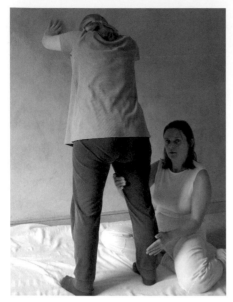

Figure 6.27 Meridian stroking of the legs.

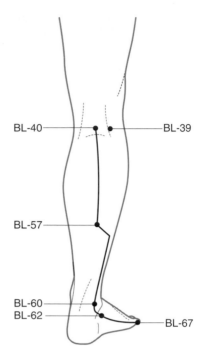

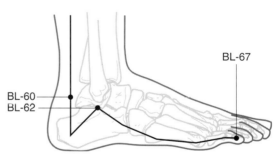

Figure 6.28 The Bladder meridian and points in the back of the leg.

moving all the meridian energy. It can also be done lightly.

Why? This stimulates all the meridians in the legs and focuses on their direction in the traditional meridian system. It can be very useful during labour itself if the mother is feeling tired, and particularly if her legs are feeling wobbly.

Caution: don't work directly over areas of varicose veins.

Palming the Bladder meridian in the legs

The previous technique is more dispersing. Palming is a more tonifiying technique.

Place the mother hand on the mother's sacrum, and with your other hand palm down the centre of the back of the mother's legs, staying on each point for as long as you feel you need to (Fig. 6.28). When you get to the knee, you may need to move the mother hand to the knee so that you can palm down the lower leg. You can follow this by working with the thumbpad in specific points. Finish by holding the foot, allowing the energy to settle.

Why? You are working the Bladder meridian. Energy flow often gets stuck here which affects the ability of the legs to support the body. This work will relieve pain down the back of the legs, whether related to the calf or thigh, or stemming

from the back such as sciatica. Bladder relates to fear and palming the meridian in the legs can help with grounding and calming.

More complex techniques (and specific points)

Bladder 39 and 40 (BL-39 and BL-40)

BL-40 lies in the back of the knee in the popliteal crease in a depression between the tendons of the muscles of biceps femoris and semitendinosus. BL-39 is to the lateral side of BL-40 and in the depression medial to biceps femoris (Fig. 6.28).

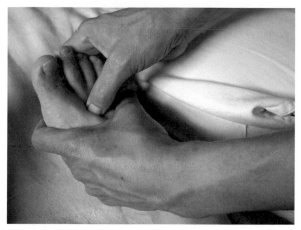

Figure 6.29 Working a specific point – note the position of the mother hand around the foot to give support to the working thumb, in this case on LV-3.

Both of these points are useful for difficulty with urination. They can be used in pregnancy as well as during labour and postnatally.

Bladder 57 (BL-57)

BL-57 (Fig. 6.28) lies midway between BL-40 and BL-60 (which is between the outer tip of the ankle bone and the achilles tendon) in the depression below the bellies of the gastrocnemius. It relaxes the calf and heel and also helps to treat haemorrhoids.

Other specific points which may be used in labour

When you are deciding to focus on a specific point, place your thumb in it and support this working thumb with the fingers of the hand (Fig. 6.29). Find a place to put the mother hand which is fairly close to the point you are working, and give support with it while working the point.

Points which may be used in pregnancy as well as labour

Why? All of these points potentially have an effect on pain relief in labour as well as other specific uses which are indicated with the point description.

Bladder 67 (BL-67)

This is on the lateral side of the base of the little toe nail. It has the effect of promoting downward movement of the head of the fetus, especially when followed by BL-60 (Fig. 6.28). This is the point that is used to turn breech babies (usually with moxa, a Chinese herb). Warming techniques are also effective to use. Rub the point as well as holding it. A good time to start is from 32 weeks. The mother can work it herself as often as she can, but only while she knows the baby is breech. If the baby turns and the point is worked again, it may turn the baby back.

Case study 6.5   Turning a breech baby – a community midwife

W attended my parentcraft classes at work. When she was 36 weeks pregnant it was confirmed that the baby was in breech. The doctors had recommended that she have an external cephalic version (ECV) to turn the baby and a date was to be booked for 2 weeks hence. As ECV is not without risks and not always effective anyway, I talked to the class about alternative methods, in particular shiatsu and moxibustion. I knelt before W and held her feet, awaiting her breathing to slow and the initial contact to be comfortable. Then I pinpointed BL-67. The baby immediately became very active and of course, the class was impressed! I did not have time to continue during the class but I suggested that she explain to her partner and see what happens at home.

A week later, W was attending my clinic. I saw that the baby was breech and spent a longer time working on BL-67 and BL-60. I also demonstrated with W several exercises associated with shiatsu, especially rocking and stretching the spine in a relaxed position. W telephoned me to say the baby had turned and when she went to the hospital to see the doctors, they were pleased to inform her that they could recommend she continue for a normal delivery.

W saw me each week at the clinic and continued to carry out the exercise, resulting in a normal delivery of a healthy infant at full term.

Kidney 1 (KI-1)

It is just below the centre of the ball of the foot, in a depression formed when the foot is plantar flexed (Fig. 6.30).

This point is known as the bubbling spring and is the only point on the sole of the foot – thus it is the lowest point on the body. As the lowest point, it links in to earth energy and is said to help the body absorb the Yin energy of the earth. In this respect it is a very calming point. As the first point of the Kidney channel, it has an effect on the whole Kidney meridian and is especially useful for drawing Kidney energy down. It can also be good in cases of exhaustion. It is the wood point

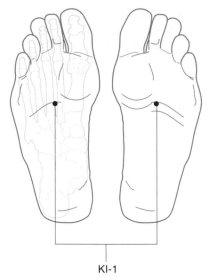

Figure 6.30   KI-1 point in the foot.

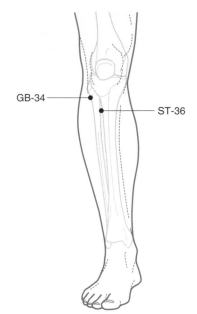

Figure 6.31   Points GB-34 and ST-36.

on the Kidney channel and therefore is helpful for balancing water and wood energies – the two main energies involved in labour.

Gall Bladder 34 (GB-34)

This lies close to Stomach 36 (ST-36). It is below the outside of the knee in the depression about 1 thumbwidth below and to the front of the head of the fibula (Fig. 6.31). It is a little bit above and to the outside of ST-36.

It is known as the 'Gathering point of the sinews', and one of its effects is to help dilate a scarred or tight cervix.

Stomach 36 (ST-36)

This lies in the groove beside the shin bone, one fingerwidth below the knob at the top of the shin-bone, i.e. the anterior crest of the tibia (Fig. 6.31). To find it, locate GB-34 first and it is one thumb-width below that point and one fingerwidth lateral to the anterior crest of the tibia. You can also slide your thumb against the tibia from below the knee. Where it stops, i.e. just below the crest of the tibia, is the point.

It has a strong effect on tonifying Ki and nour-ishing Blood and Yin energy. It can be used in almost any case of exhaustion or stuck energy. It balances earth energy and is grounding and set-tling. It is not an exaggeration to say that this is one of the most important points in the body and can be useful for almost anything. Indeed, Qin Cheng-zu of the Song dynasty wrote nearly a thousand years ago that by using it 'all diseases can be treated'.

Along with BL-60, this point helps relax the vaginal area which is good for pain relief and aids dilation. Care must be taken to check that it isn't shortening the length of the contractions, and other points should be chosen if this is the case.

Leg points which are contraindicated in pregnancy

Bladder 60, Spleen 6, Liver 3   All of these three points may be good for strengthening con-tractions, either for inducing or augmenting labour and discharging the placenta. They should not be used in pregnancy, except for induction, as they could over-stimulate the uterus. Having said that, many Japanese midwives and shiatsu practi-tioners do use them, especially Spleen 6, during the last few weeks of pregnancy to prepare a mother for going into labour. I never used to use them until at least term plus one, but in the past few years have used them from about 38 weeks in moderation, as I find they help focus the mother's energy on labour and can ease those niggly aches and pains of the last few weeks. To induce labour they tend to have to be worked quite vigorously.

Do bear in mind that each person is going to respond differently to the different points – some may cause a mother to feel a contraction almost instantaneously, others may need to be worked for at least 3–4 min for any effect, others may have no effect at all. It depends also on how far away the woman is from going into labour. The points can only focus the energy which is there. I often find that the women who don't respond to the points, don't respond to prostaglandins or low doses of syntocinon either. In labour they can also be good for pain relief as they allow the energy of the uterus to flow – but you need to be careful that they are not over-stimulating contractions.

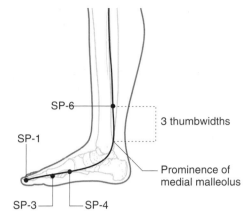

Figure 6.32   Points SP-6 and SP-1.

Case study 6.6   Labour shiatsu – induction – a community midwife

F was sitting on the antenatal ward at 9.00 am. She was overdue and agreed to have an induction. She had been contracting very mildly and irregularly overnight. On examination she had a Bishop Score of 7 and was therefore suitable for an artificial rupture of membranes. F was keen to have the baby born and agreed to transfer to a labour room for this to be carried out. The monitoring of the baby's heart was commenced and showed a normal trace. However, when the waters were broken it was noted that there was light meconium present. This can be a sign of fetal distress but is also common with overdue babies. The doctors were informed and agreed to allow labour to progress with monitoring and would review a need to augment if progress was slow.

F was now contracting 2 every 10 min and the baby's head was high. Using shiatsu with her consent I concentrated on GB-21 to encourage descent of the presenting part. To alleviate anxiety I worked on GB-20 and BL-10 on her head. She was very receptive and particularly commented on a surge of energy when GV-15 was worked on. I encouraged F to breathe slowly, out into the abdomen. Although we had to monitor the baby, F was able to sit out onto a birthing ball, suitably covered, and I was able to get to GB-34 and LV-3 whilst working on her legs and feet. She had oedema on her feet so I used a gentle stroking technique in these areas (this was to encourage contractions) and by 1.00 pm she was contracting 3 every 10 min and the contractions were strong.

By 2.00 pm F was anxious and distressed and demanding pain relief. With support using shiatsu, F got through this transitional period and delivered her baby at 4.46 pm with a minimal blood loss.

All support given during labour has proved very effective, so much so that the doctors have made a point of asking me not to use shiatsu in their studies into inductions as they believe in the effectiveness of my work!

What was striking in these cases was the ease with which the baby went to the breast and the subsequent total contentment of the baby.

F expressed her appreciation of shiatsu for childbirth.

Bladder 60   This lies between the posterior border of the external malleolus and the medial aspect of tendo calcaneus, at the same level as the tip of malleolus, i.e. in the hollow midway between the knob of the ankle bone on the outside of the ankle and Achilles tendon (Fig. 6.28).

This point is the fire point on the Bladder meridian and has the useful effect of clearing heat and excess energy, especially from the head. Because of its relationship with the Heart, it can be used for pain in the heart both physically and emotionally and can calm an anxious woman in labour. It activates the whole length of the Bladder meridian and can ease tightness in the head, spine and legs. It has a strong downward effect and so is very useful for inducing and augmenting labour and for the expulsion of the placenta.

Spleen 6 and Liver 3   These can be incorporated in foot and ankle massage. They help speed the birth of the baby.

Spleen 6 (SP-6)   Place the tip of your little finger on top of the inside ankle bone of the opposite leg, fingers pointing to the front of the leg. SP-6 lies beneath the second joint of the forefinger, under the shin, i.e. 3 cun above the tip of the medial malleolus just posterior to the tibial border (Fig. 6.32). To work the point, you need to hook up and under the bone.

This is an important point for maternity applications as well as digestive, sexual, urinary problems and emotional balancing. Although it is on the Spleen meridian, it is where Spleen meets

Liver and Kidney and so affects all these energies, i.e. earth, wood and water. All three are important in labour. It has extremely wide applications and can be used for anything to do with deficiency of Ki, Blood, Yin, Yang or Kidney Essence, failure of Spleen Ki to hold the blood in the vessels, too much Ki, Blood or dampness. It really is worth trying at any stage of labour, including induction. It can help change fetal position and is useful for regulating uterine bleeding.

Liver 3 (LV-3)   This is on top of the foot between the first and second toes, i.e. between the first and second metatarsal bones, 1.5 or 2 cun proximal to the margin of the web (Fig. 6.32). Place your finger on the space between the two bones and slide towards the ankle. It is in the depression before the junction of the bases of the first and second metatarsals. To work this point, you need to angle straight down towards the sole of the foot.

This point is very good for clearing wood energy – both by bringing more energy into the Liver or taking excess energy away. The emotion associated with wood is anger and when any emotions are suppressed then it is wood energy that gets stuck. It can help women release suppressed emotions and feel more in touch with what they are feeling in labour. Suppressed emotions are often what block the movement from first to second stage. It can therefore be a good point for transition. It can help draw energy down from where wood energy tends to get stuck in the shoulders and so is helpful for headaches. It is often useful if the mother finds the neck and shoulder points too intense. This point has an antispasmodic effect on the cervix, so it is useful in cases where the cervix is tense and not dilating with contractions.

Case study 6.7   Shiatsu for labour – a community midwife

I was called in to care for a client on the labour ward. She had arrived to be induced as she was 2 weeks post-dates. This was her first pregnancy and she was anxious, though accompanied by her supportive partner. She was 19 years old and did not know about shiatsu, which I explained to her as a form of finger-pressure acupuncture, similar to massage. She agreed to my using this as appropriate.

On examination at 0900 she had a Bishops Score of 7 and was therefore suitable for artificial rupture of membranes rather than prostaglandin gel. There was meconium grade I liquor present and the head was −3 to the ischial spines. She was not contracting for the first hour.

Initially I used the point GB-21 on the shoulder to encourage the head to engage fully, descending to a point where contractions may be encouraged. She began to contract 2:10 mildly.

I then asked her to sit out of the bed, using points GB-20 and B-10, supporting her forehead with the 'mother hand'. I did this as she was extremely anxious and I needed to encourage her to relax and mobilize. In fact, her contractions became 3:10 moderate strength and she closed her eyes and appeared to be very calm and resting, which surprised the registrar when he called later to see if she needed further augmentation.

After 2 h she said she was exhausted and appeared to become distressed. I used Governing Vessel 20 on the top of her head to help her to energize. This, together with deep breathing out into the abdomen, worked for a further 2 h. I left the room to compute notes of her admission, etc., and have a tea, leaving her with her partner. When I returned she was in tears, asking for pain relief. I explained the alternatives, examined her,

finding she was 6 cm dilated. We agreed to a Pethidine injection as I felt this would be enough to offset her immediate distress and would wear off before the second stage. This was done effectively. I stayed with her from this point, using the points Spleen 6 on the ankle, Liver 3 near the big toe to encourage labour, as contractions were slackening, and Large Intestine 4 on the thumb to offset nausea. She was also oedematous on her feet and legs and I used gentle stroking technique towards the knee.

Her baby was born at 4.46 pm by spontaneous vaginal delivery. I gave her syntometrine intramuscular injection to encourage separation of the placenta as she and her partner insisted on it – all her friends had had it. The estimated blood loss was 100 ml and she breastfed her baby immediately on delivery. No suturing was required.

On the postnatal ward I enquired as to whether she found the shiatsu helpful. She said she had, and her partner was impressed.

The medical staff and my colleagues noted that this had taken place and were amazed at the initial impact of shiatsu.

I was confident in the favourable outcome of this method of support and extremely proud that others had witnessed it. I realized that I should have had more success if I had involved her partner more in the use of shiatsu and resolved to do this on future occasions.

I hope now to introduce the theory of shiatsu to antenatal women, particularly at booking and then at parentcraft when hopefully partners will be present. I will keep records of its use and inform colleagues at a suitable midwife forum.

Arms and hands

The arms, like the legs and feet, represent the extension of energy outwards and points around the hands have a deep internal effect. While we could say that the legs relate more to earth energy of grounding, the arms relate more to the fire element and its energy of communication and connecting with others. When there is sudden shock or trauma, fire energy may get out of balance and working with it can help calm anxiety and panic. The arms also relate to the taking in of air energy through the Lungs. The ability to breathe deeply is important in labour.

Box 6.9   Lung visualization – baby breathing

This is a useful exercise for mothers to do both in pregnancy and labour. Breathe out into the hara/abdomen. Feel the movement of the breath as you breathe out and in (like the hara breathing). Gradually be more aware of your baby in your womb and feel the breath surrounding your baby's body. With each out-breath, feel the space around your baby's body. After a while, feel your breath moving within your baby's body. Be aware of how your breath is supporting your baby. Be aware of oxygen flowing in your baby's blood. Be more aware of your baby's body as separate from you but nourished by you. Now begin to be aware of your body from your baby's perspective – surrounding their body, being a limit for their movements, a boundary around them. After a while, be more aware of the movement of your breath in your body, the rise and fall of your abdomen. Place your hands over your abdomen and be aware of your baby.

Cervix breathing
In labour only, the mother can focus the movement of breath going down into the cervix and opening it up with each breath.

Often the mother does not want her arms worked on in labour because she tends to be more curled around or leaning over – going inwards and protecting herself physically and emotionally. Sometimes she may find the hand-over-hand stroking technique (stroking down over the arms from the shoulders) can help release Jitsu from the shoulders. Holding the hands, like the feet, is calming. If she is lying in a bed, in a less instinctive and more open position, she may need you to work her arms with other techniques which I cover in the pregnancy section.

More complex techniques (and specific points)

These are worked in the same way as holding specific leg points (page 111).

Heart Protector 8 (HP-8)

This is in the centre of the palm of the hand, where the tip of the middle finger lands when a fist is made (Fig. 6.33). It is said to be the mirror of Kidney 1 on the feet. Linked with the energy of the heart and fire, it has the effect of calming the emotions. It can be very good if the mother is feeling panicky and uneasy. It can be useful if the mother is not feeling comfortable in her environment, or is feeling disconnected from her baby.

Heart Protector 6 (HP-6)

This is 2 cun from the wristfold in between the two tendons (Fig. 6.33). The median nerve is under this point and therefore it should not be worked too deeply. It is calming, but is also useful for nausea and sickness in labour.

Ikuyo wrote about how holding the mother's hand would often help her to relax. She might hold or she might rub. She said that it 'warms the

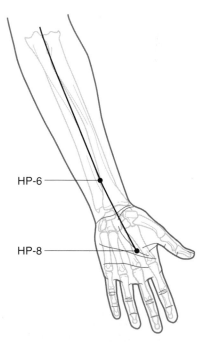

Figure 6.33   Points HP-8 and HP-6.

heart, relaxes the mother and helps her feel more calm and secure'.

Hand point not for use in pregnancy – Large intestine 4 (LI-4)

This is a point like Bladder 60, Spleen 6, Liver 3 and Gall Bladder 21 which can bring labour on and therefore should not be used in pregnancy. It is known as the great eliminator and is often used to relieve pain. It is especially useful if the mother is feeling sick or has diarrhoea.

It lies between the thumb and forefinger on the back of the hand (Fig. 6.34). To locate, either (a) have the thumb and index finger closed and the point is at the highest spot of the muscle; or (b)

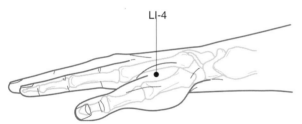

Figure 6.34 Large intestine 4.

stretch the thumb and the index finger. The point is midway between the junction of the first and second metacarpal bones and the border of the web, slightly towards the second metacarpal bone.

To work the point, move your working hand as though you are shaking the mother's hand but bringing the area between your thumb and index finger into the area between the mother's thumb and index finger. Place your thumb over the point and angle at approximately 45° into the 'v' between the bones.

Box 6.10   Exercise – opening your hands

Tighten your hands by clenching your fingers and drawing them to the centre of your palm. Notice what happens to your breathing and to your pelvis. Now open out your hands and relax them. Focus on the point in the centre of the palm (HP-8) and feel like you are breathing out through here. You can imagine that your hand is like a flower opening.

This is very useful in labour for anxiety and also for opening up the cervix. If the hand is held clenched up, this blocks the flow of energy in the rest of the body, including the cervix. You may have heard of getting women to hold combs as a pain distraction technique. From a shiatsu point of view, this is not a good idea because it is blocking the flow of energy.

Case study 6.8   Integrating shiatsu into maternity care – a community midwife

I am a community midwife working in a team of six, providing total care to a caseload of women throughout their confinement. I was on-call when H paged to say that she was in labour, first baby, term plus 6. Her labour had started 2 days ago with irregular contractions. However, her contractions had become regular and painful for the past 2 h and she was thinking of having some form of pain relief as she was getting tired.

I met H and her partner M in the delivery suite. I had already met H during her pregnancy twice and spoken on the phone a couple of times, so already knew her a little. On admission, H's vital signs and baby's heart tracing were within the norm expected. On internal examination her cervix was 4 cm dilated and the presenting part engaged. The membranes ruptured spontaneously during the examination.

H had a birth plan which included an epidural for pain relief so I thought she wouldn't be amenable to complementary therapy to ease her labour, but she said that she would try to manage for as long as she could. Her contractions had become irregular and less strong following admission so I suggested to H that she mobilized to encourage the presenting part to descend

and stimulate contractions; but H declined as she felt tired and wanted to rest.

I suggested a foot massage to help H relax and worked some shiatsu and reflexology points. I am not sure if it was the massage/acupressure or just nature taking its course, but H's contractions became regular and within an hour she was requesting an epidural. However, the anaesthetist was busy in the operating theatre with an emergency Caesarean section and so meanwhile I commenced H on Entonox and suggested she turn on 'all fours' as she was not comfortable on her back and it would also enable me to massage her back. The top of the bed was raised and I tucked in a bean bag for H to lean over. M was supporting her in the front and I encouraged him to massage H's shoulders as she was all hunched up. I remembered the Gall Bladder 21 point on the top of the shoulders, which is supposed to have a descending effect, and got M to massage the shoulder area while I began giving light massage to H's sacral area. Her pain was mainly in the suprapubic area and as labour progressed I also applied thumb pressure to the sacral grooves as well as alternating with leaning with my palms down on the sacral area. H said it felt good to have pressure on that area. It is an instinctive thing I do and by learning more about shiatsu I now think in terms of Chi flowing through meridians which, when stagnant (Jitsu) or deficient (Kyo), could cause problems for a person's well-being. The flow of Chi is encouraged by the application of pressure to meridian points to 'move' the stagnation or 'tonify' the deficiency to bring relief.

The anaesthetist was still unavailable due to another emergency and it was over an hour since H had first requested an epidural. Luckily she was still coping with her labour, but I felt I was failing to give her what she had planned. I compensated by giving all my energy to do what I could to ease her pain. As she was still kneeling over the head of the bed, I realized that her ankles were neatly propped up and I could work on them. I remembered that there were points around the malleolus that would help with pain relief and taught M to continue the sacral massage whilst I was doing that.

I got an intravenous drip going in anticipation for the anaesthetist but she was still busy. Anyway, I realized that labour may be progressing well as H was beginning to breathe differently and making some grunting noises. It was at this stage that the anaesthetist became available. I thought I had better examine H prior to any intervention and I couldn't believe it but H was nearly fully dilated and the baby's head had descended well into the pelvis. H felt she was really 'going somewhere' and we said 'no thank you' to the epidural. It had only taken 3 h for H to reach this stage. A baby boy weighing 7 lb 8 oz was delivered after 35 min of second stage. H and M were jubilant and couldn't belief that she had a literally 'drug free' labour. Not by choice! But it turned out so well.

I must admit that my experience in using complementary therapies as part of the care to the women I look after is limited at present. However, this case has given me confidence to realize that labour can be managed differently. I just can't wait for my next case.

I saw H on the postnatal ward the following day and we had a chance to debrief. I was worried that H may be upset that she did not have an epidural as she had wanted. H said she felt that the contractions were painful but it was bearable. She said that the work I was doing on her back was comforting and the fact that I was there beside her was important.

H is really pleased with her care and she said she felt very proud of herself for coping with her labour without drugs. That is empowerment.

I am very excited that I can offer alternative care to women in childbirth. I feel that though childbirth is very much medicalized it can work 'hand in hand' with complementary therapies to enable women to have the best of both worlds.

Point combinations

Combining points is about bringing two different energies together. There are some useful point combinations in labour – although potentially any two points can be linked. You don't necessarily have to stick to these combinations – you can try any others which you feel are helpful for the particular mother you are working with. Use whichever thumb pads or finger tips are most comfortable for you and make sure that you have good mother-hand support with the rest of the hand. Work points on both sides of the body.

Ikuyo Hosaka's point combinations

Ikuyo often used point combinations in her work.

'The magic triangle'

Ikuyo often referred to the 'magic triangle'. This is SP-6, BL-60 and a point on the Gall Bladder which we have not been able to identify precisely but is either GB-37, 38 or 39 or may even be all three depending on different women. GB-38 is 4 thumbwidths above the tip of the outside ankle bone at the anterior border of the fibula, GB-37 is 5 cun above GB-39 and 3 thumbwidths above the tip of the outside ankle bone between the posterior border of the fibula and the tendons of peroneus longus and brevis (Fig. 6.35). None are specified particularly for induction, but all are indicated for alleviating pain. This combination is useful for inducing labour and augmenting contractions.

Three points on the foot

Ikuyo would often combine LV-3 and KI-1 with GB-43 (Fig. 6.36). GB-43 is between the fourth toe and the little toe, 0.5 thumbwidth in from the margin of the web.

She found that if this was done in early labour then the mother wouldn't get cramp.

Other suggestions

Joining above and below

It is often useful if you have two people working to combine LV-3 with GB-21 – GB-21 sends wood energy down and LV-3 draws wood energy down. This is very useful as a focus to stimulate second-stage contractions.

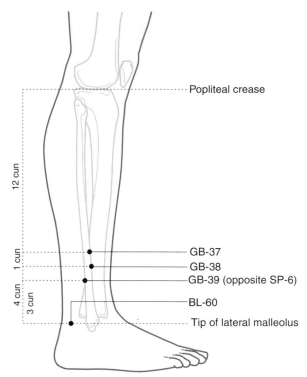

Figure 6.35   Points of the magic triangle: SP-6, BL-60 and GB-37–GB-39.

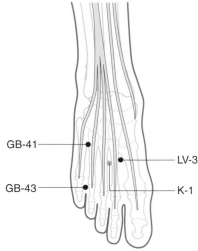

Figure 6.36   Combined points on the foot: LV-3, KI-1, GB-41 and GB-43.

Hand and foot elimination

LV-3 and LI-4 is another point combination. This helps with elimination and letting go, and helps the individual actions of the points be more effective.

Please refer to Appendix 3 for further information on matters relating to safety and diagnosis issues.

Case study 6.9   By a senior hospital midwife

This gives a good idea of how shiatsu can be used in more complicated cases alongside conventional treatments and with careful monitoring.

G, age 42, had a past obstetric history of five previous full-term normal vaginal deliveries with uncomplicated pregnancies. All her children are now in their teens. She also had a past medical history of depression requiring treatment. In 1999 she had a malignant polyp in the anal canal removed, and was given the 'all clear' for cancer last August.

She became pregnant in April. This was an unplanned pregnancy but the family were happy and looking forward to the birth. In June, constant lower abdominal pain prompted an urgent referral to the specialist who confirmed that there was an abdominal mass which was most likely to be a recurrence of malignancy. G, after consultation with the cancer specialist, opted to continue with the pregnancy until the baby was mature enough to be delivered and to have surgery and chemotherapy if appropriate after delivery. She was admitted to hospital when she was 30 weeks pregnant because she needed strong painkillers in the form, firstly of pethidine and, later when this was ineffective, of morphine. When she was 34 weeks, she developed bilateral deep vein thrombosis which required an intravenous infusion of

heparin, a blood-thinning drug. She and her baby were closely monitored.

The pregnancy progressed until 35 weeks when a decision was made to deliver the baby. This was because of the concern about the adverse side effects of long-term use of morphine on the baby. Once the baby was delivered G would be able to continue with cancer treatment. Careful consideration was made as to the type of induction to use because of the high number of previous pregnancies – she was considered to be at high risk because of this.

The plan was to give G one dose of 1 mg prostin gel the next day and attempt to help dilate the cervix enough, in order to rupture the membranes. She had a further four doses of prostin on 4 consecutive days. On day 6 she was seen and examined by the consultant obstetrician who artificially ruptured the membranes. She did not have any contractions after this procedure. On day 7 she was started on an oxytocin drip at 9.30 am. She was only contracting very irregularly when I attended at 12.50 pm. G was on a PCA pump of a narcotic called fentanyl for pain relief.

This was making her nauseous and she had vomited a few times which was causing her some distress. She

was given two different types of antiomotic. Although I
wasn't her main carer, I knew about G and her history
and had spoken to her a few times in passing. I was very
keen to try the techniques I had learnt recently to help G,
not just to get her into labour but also to support and help
her with pain. She was very demoralized as well because
of the length of time she had spent on the labour ward.
After explaining to G and her mother and best friend who
were also in the delivery room about shiatsu, I obtained
G's verbal consent to proceed.

I placed my mother (right) hand on the uterus (lower
part) and my left hand on her chest over her heart. This
was done firstly to achieve a connection with G's body.
As I focused my mind on my 'hara' and on my inhalation
and exhalation, I could sense that she was Jitsu in the
chest area and Kyo in the uterus, so I slowly palmed my
left hand down to the abdominal area. She felt a sense
that there was less tightness in the chest after a few
repetitions. Next, I used HP-6, applying perpendicular
thumb pressure alternating between both of her hands to
relieve her of the nausea. This was very effective. I also
worked on the kidney/uterus connection by placing my
left hand on the kidney area and right hand on the
uterus. This was just a placing of hands – no pressure
was applied and I kept my hands in this position for a few
breaths. I felt that she needed to have the kidney energy
diverted to the uterus. My next approach was with my
right hand on the left kidney and my left on the right; I
gently palmed my hands bringing them together in the
uterus area. This was very well received by G. My next
approach was on governing vessel 20. After only
applying thumb pressure once, I abandoned this area
because G felt very dizzy. I felt I could work on this point
because her blood pressure was normal and GV-20
can be useful in dilatation of the cervix. I then proceeded
to work on GB-21 and LI-4, alternating between these
points. I started at 12.50 and by 13.20 she was

contracting strongly about 5 every 10 min. At this point,
the oxytocin drip had to be reduced. I was able to work
on her back, particularly the lower back and sacral area,
when she turned into a kneeling position. Using the
thumb on either side of the lumbar spine I worked on the
bladder points. Stroking with both palms on either side of
the lower spine, I was able to give G a sensation of the
'opening up' of her pelvis. I left her at 14.00 in the care of
her midwife when I was confident that she was in
established labour.

I returned to review her at 15.45 when G was very
distressed with contractions and losing control. She was
extremely tired and was not getting any pain relief at all
from the PCA pump. She was begging for a Caesarean
section and an epidural. An epidural was contraindicated
in her case because of the long-term heparin use.
I decided to calm her using HP-8 and SP-4, alternating
between the right and the left side. This was very effective
in that she was clearly quite drowsy between contractions
and was able to re-focus on her breathing exercises. At
16.20 she complained of perineal pressure. She was
examined and found to be fully dilated. We encouraged
her to push. She delivered 8 min later a healthy baby girl.
The placenta was delivered easily and her baby's
breathing was not depressed, as was anticipated.

Personal reflection
The satisfaction of achieving a good outcome from the
techniques that I used in this case has boosted my
confidence immensely. G's companions who were in the
delivery room throughout her labour were also impressed
with the success of shiatsu. Verbal feedback from G was
very positive. She was very elated and animated about the
techniques I used and related this to the consultant
obstetrician in charge of her case. The support and
encouragement from my medical colleagues has given me
the impetus to persevere with using the shiatsu course.

Summary

Labour is a time when shiatsu can play a powerful role
in enabling a mother to connect with her body and
achieve a 'natural' birth. It is an opportunity for her
partner to be involved. Points and work may be done
throughout the whole of labour, if it feels appropriate
for the mother. The midwife may need to work with the
partner to offer this kind of one-to-one care.

Even when there are medical interventions, shiatsu
can continue to be used as it works with the energy of
the whole body and does not interact with drugs.

Make sure that you know the contraindicated
points for pregnancy.

Reflect on the following questions:
- Are there any techniques you already use
  which are similar to any of the shiatsu techniques?
  If so, how are they similar?
- Would you be able to integrate any of these into
  your antenatal classes?
- Do a lesson plan for an antenatal class including
  some of these ideas.
- Think about how you would teach these to
  partners during labour itself.
- Identify any training needs for learning these
  techniques and being able to teach them to
  women and their partners.

Case study 6.10 Example of integrating shiatsu in an antenatal class. 'Labour in motion' – Carol, a hospital midwife

---

'Labour in motion' is a single antenatal session I facilitate for women and their birth partners. It was created from a recognition of the need to help women to rediscover their instinctual behaviour, build confidence in their ability to birth their babies and give them an understanding of the process of birth. The aim of the session is to reduce fear, encourage mobility in labour, reduce interventions and to help women to achieve the best possible birth.

Each 'Labour in motion' session lasts around two and half hours and includes:

- A description of labour, shared coping strategies, an explanation of the reason for the pain of labour and how to work with the pain.
- A simple relaxation and breath technique (re-learning relaxed abdominal breathing and focusing on a slow out-breath).
- Positions for labour and birth.
- Optimal fetal positioning, including the benefits of kneeling and crawling, and a demonstration of the 'cat' yoga position.
- A short meditation of visualizing the baby.
- A demonstration and practical application of some simple massage. This includes teaching the partners how to stroke down the Bladder meridian, to use thumb pressure along the Bladder and Kidney meridians and the value of working on the sacrum in labour. I suggest working with the breath, working from the hara, the importance of intention and feedback, and the need for practice; also that they try to visualize the baby coming down.

I take a pelvis into the session. With the aid of the pelvis, I can show the couples the position of the sacral foramen and emphasize the importance of not putting direct pressure on the spine. I also advise them not to use too much pressure on the sacrum during pregnancy. During their practice in the session, I work around the couples, helping them find what feels right to them. I hope that the sessions improve communication between the couples and that the result will be enhanced support for the woman in labour. I believe that incorporating aspects of shiatsu into the sessions helps to create balance and a holistic approach, which enhances the preparation of women and their partners for labour.

Techniques to teach (women and their birth partners) parents for labour in an antenatal class

---

It depends how much time you have to show things. Carol gives an example of one session.

I run two two and a half hour sessions or a 1 day workshop. Pregnant women attend the sessions with their birth partner/s about 1–3 months before the due date.

Theory – I keep this very simple. I tend not to refer to Kyo and Jitsu, but simply to get people to feel the different qualities of energy and to learn to tune in to how long to stay and how deeply to work. The birth partner/s only have to learn how to work with one person – and that one person can give good feedback. I explain that shiatsu is working the same points and meridians as acupuncture, and that the work will have both a physical and emotional effect. I talk about how the mother's and baby's energy is interlinked.

Practical techniques
Demonstration of some of the basic principles – pressure, breathing, working from the hara (which I tend to call the abdomen or belly) and having the shoulders relaxed, through integrating the shiatsu with breathing and showing the abdominal holding and the general abdominal pressures. This gives an opportunity for the woman and partner/s to connect with the baby.

Stroking of the Girdle Vessel – stroking and holding on the Governing Vessel and Bladder, explaining why and when this would be useful but not talking specifically about the function of the meridian.

The induction points – getting the mother to work on the partner/s i.e. SP-6, LV-3, GB-21, BL-60 and LI-4. If there is time, I also show the calming points HP-8 and KI-1 foot.

Work on the neck and shoulders – BL-10 and GB-20 and shoulder leaning, and work with GB-21.

REFERENCES

Masunaga S 1977 Zen shiatsu. Japan Publications, Tokyo

Pitchford P 1993 Healing with whole foods, oriental traditions and modern nutrition. North Atlantic Books, Berkeley, California, USA

Sutton J, Scott P 1995 Understanding and teaching optimal foetal positioning. Birth concepts. Tauranga, New Zealand

7

Shiatsu for pregnancy and the early postnatal period

Introduction

Pregnancy is when a midwife trained in shiatsu skills will probably work differently from a shiatsu practitioner – not only because the midwife will not be doing a full diagnosis, but because she will not have as much time to work. I have included some longer sequences for the midwife who can spend more time with a mother, but I have also included short sequences, even a few point combinations, if the midwife only has 5 or 10 min. It can still be effective to work for short spaces of time. This is often how shiatsu is used in Japan, as a first aid measure.

Case study 7.1   Midwife shiatsu practitioner working with a pregnant woman

L worked with a 41-year-old client with two young children, both home births.

She came at 27 weeks feeling very tired and stiff (especially in her hips and shoulders) and with pain in her sacro-iliac joint. My impression was that her depleted water was unable to control her wood energy, resulting in J being stuck in her wood and consequently very stiff and uncomfortable. Initial treatments mainly tonified depleted kidney and moved stagnated GB and LI.

Each treatment involved spending time holding the kidney diagnostic area and treating BL-23 and GV-4 to tonify her kidney energy. I feel working CV may have also helped to strengthen the kidneys by circulating Essence.

Much of the work also concentrated on her sacrum and buttocks, using strong work to release the stuck energy. During the early sessions there was little change in the energy patterns and shiatsu only provided short-term relief of J's symptoms. I have to say that I felt quite despondent about this and decided, on the advice of Suzanne Yates, to focus more on the sacrum, BL in the legs and the Girdle Vessel. I also spent longer holding the opening and associated points to balance the energy rather than for diagnosis only. Slowly, the kidney energy became stronger and by the fourth session the wood energy had moved into fire and metal, allowing J to let go of her stiffness. Consequently, the sacro-iliac joint pain improved.

On reflection, work on earth to support and strengthen water may have been appropriate, as well as more work on opening the chest and lung to enable Ki to be taken into the body and taken down to the kidneys. It may also have been useful to spend some time balancing the three burners.

The feedback from J was that she found the shiatsu very relaxing. After each session she felt very exhausted for the rest of the day, which made her rest. Usually the following couple of days she felt more energized. She also felt that it helped her general stiffness and consequently the sacro-iliac joint pain.

Techniques for pregnancy

Many of the techniques which are useful in labour can be used antenatally, especially in the second and third trimester, as well as postnatally. You need to know the points which are not safe to use in pregnancy until term, or for facilitating induction.

Box 7.1   Summary of induction points

These are all points which have a strong effect on the Uterus. They are good for stimulating or augmenting labour but should not be used in pregnancy, apart from to induce labour.

- Legs/Feet – Spleen 6, Liver 3, Bladder 60
- Shoulder – Gall Bladder 21
- Hand – Large Intestine 4

You need to bear in mind that even those points which are safe to use tend to be worked much less vigorously and for less time. The abdomen is important to work throughout the pregnancy, although during the first trimester the techniques will be more of the gentler holding ones, rather than specific points. You may find you can combine these while doing abdominal palpations. The idea of incorporating the mother hand into your palpations with the aim of giving support, either from the back or another place on the abdomen, can help the mother feel more reassured. Try it and see any differences. You could also use palpation as a time to connect the mother with her breathing and to do whatever other abdominal or lower back work that feels appropriate such as Girdle Vessel or Heart–Uterus, Kidney–Uterus.

The strong sacrum and lower back techniques of labour are not suitable for the first trimester, when the focus is on allowing energy to gather in the uterus rather than moving energy too much. By the middle of the second trimester, when the pregnancy is established, then this work can be very useful for alleviating lower backache. Neck and shoulder work is useful throughout pregnancy – avoiding the induction point in the shoulder (Gall Bladder 21).

The mother's position for these techniques depends on the context in which you see her. Traditionally, shiatsu is done lying on the floor, using mainly the supine, prone or side position. The prone position is not usually comfortable after the first trimester and so the side position is used instead. However, as with labour, you can work in any position. If you want to encourage a posterior baby to turn, then you may well want the mother in the all fours position. In a clinic situation, you may want the mother in a sitting position, either in a chair or propped up on a bed with cushions. If you are visiting the mother in her home, you have the additional option of using a duvet or blankets on the floor. If you have bad knees it is easier for you if the mother is not on the ground. What is most important is to apply the basic principles.

Abdominal work

This is a way of helping the mother to begin to feel in touch with her baby. It is deeply relaxing, helps deepen the breathing and tends to settle the energy. This is some of the most valuable work to do throughout the pregnancy.

Basic techniques

You can use the labour techniques such as abdominal holding, Kidney–Uterus and Girdle Vessel (pages 105–107). Kidney–Uterus is good if the mother is exhausted or the baby is not growing well. Girdle Vessel is good for supporting the pelvis – especially if the mother has weak joints or abdominal muscles. Pressure is usually quite light in the first trimester.

Heart–Uterus The easiest way of working this is with the mother lying on her back or sitting; thus, if the mother is lying on the bed in labour, this technique can be useful. It is especially good in the first trimester.

Place one of your hands under the mother's lower back (the mother hand) over a place where it feels comfortable. Place your other hand (working hand) on her abdomen over the uterus. Focus on her out-breath and, with each out-breath, allow your hands to be drawn in more deeply. Connect with the baby – in the first trimester this will be a more energetic connection than physical. Keeping the connection with the hand on the uterus, move your hand from the back and place it over the mother's heart (Fig. 7.1). Connect deeply with her heart. Feel the heart beating, tune into its rhythm. After a while, feel which organ seems the most Kyo and which the most Jitsu. Keeping one hand (the mother hand) over the most Kyo organ, palm with the other hand to the most Jitsu. If you are not sure, then it is best to palm down from the heart to the uterus, as this is usually the direction you need to work, especially in the first trimester. Although, as pregnancy progresses the uterus will always feel physically full, energetically it may be that the heart is fuller.

If the mother is lying on her side, you may find you need to open her position by moving her upper arm back so that you can place your hand over the heart. It is easier to do with the mother lying on her right side so that her heart is uppermost.

You may find it a little more awkward if the mother has large breasts. Do what you feel comfortable with.

Why? It regulates blood/energy flow to the uterus which includes the placenta and baby, and therefore helps in all situations where there are problems with the development of either the placenta or baby. It puts the mother in touch with her emotions and her feelings of connection or lack of connection with her baby. As the energy settles and balances, it can be very calming for both mother and baby. In the first trimester, the Heart is often hot and working down can help alleviate morning sickness. If the mother is anxious about the baby's growth or movements, this can help her be more aware of what is really going on.

In labour, it can be helpful at times when the mother is feeling particularly anxious or quite flushed and hot, over-talkative, or when the baby is distressed. If the mother is not lying on her back or side, just connect as best you can.

Postnatally, it is often indicated because of the loss of Heart–Blood. It helps with postnatal depression and exhaustion.

It is a powerful connection to work with as a visualization and by getting the mother to do it herself by placing her own hands over the organs. This can be useful both in a one-to-one or class situation.

Box 7.2 Heart–Uterus visualization

Close your eyes and breathe out into your hara. When you are breathing out deeply, place both hands over your uterus and focus your attention inside your body to the uterus. Be aware of the size and shape of the uterus. Be aware of the textures of the uterus. Be aware of the size of the baby growing inside.

After a while, place one of your hands over your heart. Remember the heart is slightly to the left. Find the place where you can feel the heart beating. Feel the movement and rhythm of the heart. Get a sense of whether the heart feels warmer or cooler than the uterus.

If there is a strong difference, then you can palm with one hand moving from the warmer organ to the cooler one, imagining that you are bringing warmth to the cooler organ.

As you do this, be aware of how energy is flowing from the heart to the baby. Be aware of the flow of blood nourishing the baby. Be aware of the flow of feelings and emotions nourishing the baby.

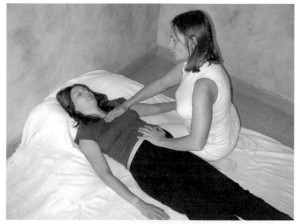

Figure 7.1 Working the Heart–Uterus.

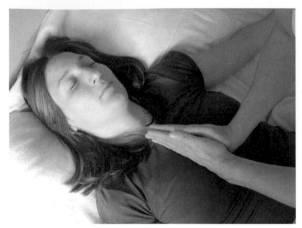

Figure 7.2   Palming along the Conception Vessel, using the side of the hands.

Palming along the Conception Vessel

Basic version With the mother lying on her back, place the little finger sides of both of your hands over the area between the centre of the breasts (Fig. 7.2). This is on the midline of the sternum, in a depression between the nipples. As the mother breathes out, lean at 90° into her body with both hands, with fairly gentle pressure. On this part of the body, the pressure is a lot less than on the sacrum and, as when working with the abdomen, it is best to start gently and get good feedback as to the amount of pressure that is comfortable. Some women are particularly sensitive here and will only like light pressure. After a few breaths, move the side of one of your hands to a short way down on the midline of the torso. You are effectively 'palming' except using the side of your hand along the midline down to as close to the pubic bone as feels comfortable. Make sure that your intention is to palm at 90° to the angle of the body. If it is later on in pregnancy, when the mother may be more propped up, you need to be aware of this angle. If you are not going in at 90° you can be pulling on the structures of the skin, which is not so comfortable.

More complex You can work along this meridian using thumb pressure. Place your mother hand over a Kyo area of the meridian and use your thumbs in either an upwards or downwards direction. There are some important points along the meridian for tonifying the uterus (see abdominal work in Chapter 6). As long as you use the right amount of pressure for each person, work in this way will be safe and appropriate.

Additional points (refer back to Fig. 6.26):

- CV-12 – midway between the umbilicus and sternocostal muscle, 4 thumbwidths above the navel. This benefits the Stomach and is used for all kinds of digestive problems including heartburn and epigastric pain.
- CV-14 – 6 thumbwidths above the navel. It benefits the Heart, calms the Shen (Spirit) and helps Lung and Stomach energy to move downwards.
- CV-17 – on the middle of the sternum. It benefits the Heart Protector, opens the chest and helps Lung and Stomach Ki to move downwards. It also benefits the breasts and promotes lactation.

Why? The Conception Vessel undergoes many changes in pregnancy, especially in the first trimester. It is important to keep energy flowing well in it to ensure a good flow of energy to the uterus, with which it connects. Usually it is best to work down it, i.e. towards the uterus, for this reason. Emotionally this can be very settling, and it will help ease feelings of nausea or heat in the upper body. Occasionally it may be indicated to work upwards, away from the uterus, to move energy up to the arms and upper body – but only do this if you are really sure that this is what is needed. An example of this can be if it feels there is too much energy in the Uterus – as for example when there are overly strong contractions and the mother is beginning to panic, or in pregnancy if there are strong pre-labour contractions.

More complex

Palming along the Penetrating Vessel/ Kidney You can use the same techniques as with the Conception Vessel ('palming' with the side of your hand and thumbing) but you need to focus on the line in the chest which is 2 thumbwidths away from the Conception Vessel and in the abdomen 0.5 thumbwidth from it (Fig. 7.3). You can also work one side at a time, or both sides at a time.

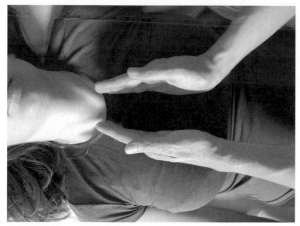

Figure 7.3 Working the Penetrating Vessel with the sides of the hands.

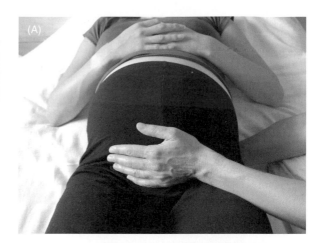

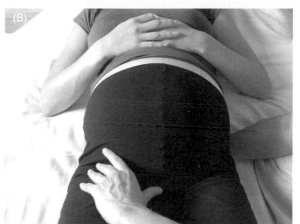

Figure 7.4 Working the pubic bone using A, the sides of the hand, and B the thumb.

Why? The Penetrating Vessel, like the Conception Vessel, undergoes many changes especially in the first trimester. It is excellent for emotional calming and easing nausea, as well as nourishing the baby and uterus. It is working with similar energies to Heart–Uterus.

Pubic bone work With your mother hand under the lower back, use the little finger side of your hand to 'palm' along the top of the pubic bone (Fig. 7.4A). You can also use thumb pressures (Fig. 7.4B).

Neck, back and side

Many changes take place in the back – the most obvious being increased lordosis of the spine. As with labour, energy tends to rise and get stuck in the neck and shoulders, especially in our culture, where women are often very sedentary during their pregnancies.

All the neck and back work shown in Chapter 6 can be beneficial for easing backaches, headaches, shoulder tension and increasing the energy of the mother. In the first trimester, it is not advisable to do strong work on the sacrum, but gentle holds and connections may feel relaxing.

The palming techniques on the Governing Vessel, Kidney and Bladder (see pages 91–92) are excellent – but, after the first trimester, will need to be done on the side or in the all fours position as in labour.

What we can add in during pregnancy are some stretches in the side-lying position, which not only work the back, but also release tension from the side of the body, where it is often stored. Stretches are not usually suitable in the first trimester, as they shift energy too much at a time when energy needs to be gathered in the uterus. They are more indicated from the second trimester and as the baby grows, when the mother feels compression in her ribs and side. This is often due to the wood energy being contracted and not able to flow. All these new techniques are more complex and need to be done by a midwife who has undergone some training, but I include them to give an idea of the type of stretching that may be suitable in pregnancy.

Case study 7.2   By a community midwife

B was expecting her first baby. When I first met her in my antenatal clinic she was well wrapped up from the cold and she said that her shoulders ached. I told her about my interest in shiatsu and that I had attended a course for midwives with Suzanne Yates in Bristol. I offered to do a quick neck and shoulder massage to help relieve her discomfort. She accepted and I massaged her trapezius muscle over her shoulders which were quite tight. After only about 5 min she appeared to relax and said that she felt more comfortable.

I saw her again at about 20 weeks of pregnancy and she was obviously in pain when she walked in. She said she had a sharp pain in her lower back, right buttock and thigh that made bending and walking very uncomfortable. After I had done the routine antenatal check she accepted a shiatsu massage on her back. I did not have much time to help her as my appointments were only for 15 min.

I worked the four sacral points BL-31–34 and did a gentle massage over her sacrum using the palm of my hand. I also suggested that she try some exercises especially on all fours and leaning forwards, including the cat stretch. She enjoyed the massage but did not immediately feel the benefit and in her own words hobbled home. The next morning she found that the pain was much more manageable and in a couple of days the pain had subsided.

A few weeks later, the pain returned and I repeated the massage showing C, her partner, what to do. The pain eased more quickly this time and did not return.

It is interesting to note that B also suffered with what the doctors thought was an overstretched uterine ligament at about 30 weeks of pregnancy. I thought she had symptoms of a uterine prolapse. On this occasion, I suggested she rested on her knees with her buttocks higher than her head to help with this; she found this position relieved her symptoms and eventually got better after a few weeks.

B had her baby daughter at 36 weeks.

Her labour was very quick and unfortunately I missed the birth as I was on holiday.

B's own account

When I was about 4 months pregnant, I started experiencing a sharp pain in my lower back, right buttock and upper leg. Bending and walking were at best very uncomfortable. My midwife explained that sciatic nerve pain was one of the numerous joys of pregnancy but she was willing to try a shiatsu massage on my lower back. At the time of the massage all I could feel were tingles running down my legs. It was comfortable and it didn't hurt to have my back rubbed. The relief was not immediate and I hobbled home without a second thought. The next morning when I woke up the pain was much more manageable and in just a couple of days the pain subsided. The discomfort reappeared after a couple of weeks but my midwife repeated the massage and again the pain disappeared, not to reappear in a couple of days. I would be willing to repeat my story should anybody want to hear it again! And obviously, I would be delighted to recommend shiatsu to anybody suffering from a similar ailment.

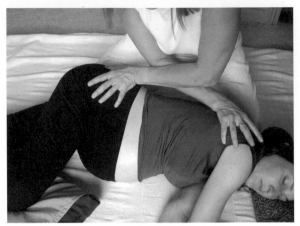

Figure 7.5   Side stretch. Note the practitioner's position with the hara facing onto the back. You need to lean directly between the two hands so as to apply even pressure.

Complex techniques

Side stretches for the back and side   All of these are done with the mother lying on her side.

Face your hara to the mother's body and cross your arms. Place one hand underneath her armpit and one hand on the hip, being careful to be below the soft tissue above the iliac crest (Fig. 7.5). Move your hara forwards so that you lean down into your hands and stretch the area of the side which is between them.

Why?   From an Eastern viewpoint, the hips and pelvis are related to the shoulders. Working one benefits the other; tightness or looseness in one area is often linked with similar or opposite in the other area. This work also relates to the Gall Bladder meridian, the main meridian for the side of the body and for regulating physical activity.

In pregnancy, there is a movement of the rib cage and compression of the side. These movements help ease this.

Neck, shoulders and spine

Shoulder and neck stretches

Kneel, sit or stand beside the mother, facing her head. Lift her upper arm and link your two hands around her shoulder, so that your fingers are on top of the shoulder (Fig. 7.6). Lean back

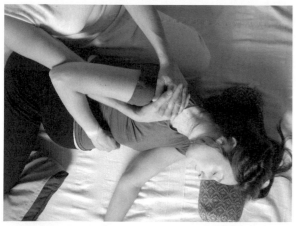

Figure 7.6   Stretching the shoulder. Note the stretch comes from the practitioner's hara moving back.

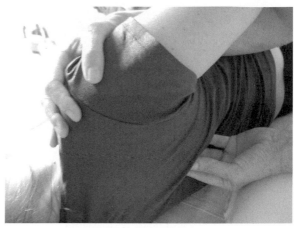

Figure 7.8   Working around the scapula.

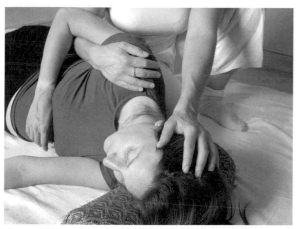

Figure 7.7   Relaxing the head. The mother hand is on the shoulder.

from your hara, keeping your arms relaxed, to open the shoulder and stretch out the neck. Repeat a few times, till you feel the area relaxing.

Relaxing the head

Keep your hand, which is nearest to the mother's body, applying slight pressure to the shoulder, and place the palm of your hand which is furthest from her body on the side of her head (Fig. 7.7). Palm down the side of the head.

Relaxing the upper back and shoulder blade

Keep the hand on the shoulder, and with the other hand palm down the upper back and around the shoulder blade.

Scapula stretch

Open the shoulder by moving it slightly away from you with the hand on the shoulder (mother hand). Place the fingers of the hand which was palming under the top of the scapula (Fig. 7.8). Draw the shoulder towards you with the mother hand so that the fingers of the working hand go deeply into the muscle. Work down and around the scapula. Repeat this sequence several times, until you feel the maximum stretch and relaxation of the muscles.

Neck work

Starting with one hand on the shoulder and one hand on the head (as in relaxing the head above), lean between the two hands to open up the side of the neck and relax the head. Refer back to Fig. 7.7.

Gall Bladder meridian

To work the Gall Bladder (GB) meridian, begin by placing one hand on the base of the skull and one hand on the shoulder and leaning between them to stretch the GB meridian.

Keeping one hand on the shoulder, begin to work with thumb pressure of the hand which was at the base of the skull (Fig. 7.9). Start at GB-20 (page 100) and work down the GB line with the thumb, to the shoulder. Avoid GB-21 in the top of the shoulder during pregnancy.

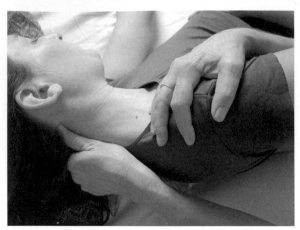

Figure 7.9 Working the Gall Bladder in the neck. Note the mother hand on the shoulder.

Bladder meridian

Move the head if necessary in order to be able to reach with your thumb the area to each side of the cervical vertebrae.

Start at BL-10 (page 99) and work with thumb pressure down each side of the cervical vertebrae, about 0.5 thumbwidth out.

Why? The neck and upper back area is related to the lower back – if there is tension/weakness in one area then there may be the corresponding, or opposite feeling in the other area.

The Gall Bladder meridian relates to hormonal changes – it can affect headaches and tension in the neck and jaw area.

For information on Bladder see page 100.

Arms

In pregnancy, the flow of energy to the arms can often be blocked by the ribs being displaced upwards and by the increasing weight of the baby pushing against the ribs. This affects the whole of the upper body, neck and shoulders, as well as the main meridians of the arms – Lung and Large Intestine, Heart and Small Intestine, Heart Protector and Triple Heater. It can cause problems with breathing (Lung energy), oedema and carpal tunnel syndrome (Lung and Triple Heater), nausea and heat rising. These are the fire–heart emotions relating to relationships, and the metal emotions of grief and re-defining identity.

The arms can be worked easily in either the side position or the supine. We can work single points,

like in labour, or the whole meridian. To work the whole meridian, if the mother was sitting, she would need to be able to have her arms supported.

Complex techniques for the arms

Heart Protector meridian Place the mother's arm nearest to you so that it is resting on the floor or bed at right angles to her body, palm up. This exposes the meridian, which is in the centre of the arm. Place your mother hand below the centre of her clavicle and with your working hand palm along the centre of the arm to her palm. You can follow this with working with your thumb pad.

The main points on this meridian are HP-6 and HP-8 which were covered in Chapter 6.

If there is oedema, it is best to work with the arm elevated to help the oedema drain.

Why? Heart Protector is closely linked to the Heart and the many changes that take place in Blood circulation (in both Eastern and Western terms), especially in the first trimester when these changes relate to the emotional ups and downs the mother experiences. It may be Heart energy rising up which causes the feeling of nausea and heat in the first trimester, and HP-6 has long been established in the treatment of nausea. The partner meridian of Triple Heater, it can help with oedema.

Lung This is worked in the same way as Heart Protector, but the arm is placed at 45° to the side of the body to expose the Lung meridian which is along the lateral edge of the arm towards the thumb (Fig. 7.10).

Why? It affects breathing and opens the chest, and is about our sense of self.

Important points To work specific points, work them as was described in Chapter 6. If you are including them as part of work on a meridian, then you can keep the mother hand still on one area and simply move the working hand to access the different points.

Lung 1 (LU-1) This is on the lateral aspect of the chest, in the interspace between the first and second ribs, 6 thumbwidths lateral to the midline of the chest (Fig. 7.11).

This point is an important point that affects the organ of the Lung. It can be used to promote easier breathing and to clear congestion from the chest.

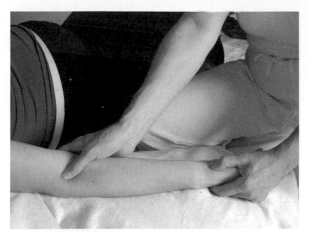

Figure 7.10   Working points on the Lung meridian. Note the position of the arm alongside the body.

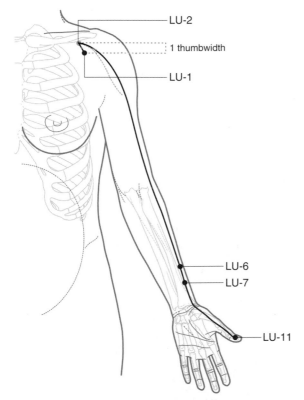

Figure 7.11   Points on the Lung meridian.

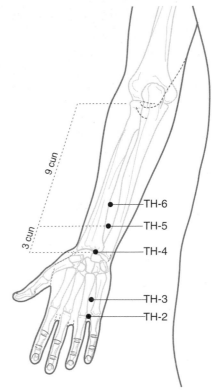

Figure 7.12   Points on the Triple Heater, TH-2–6.

It also works along with the Stomach meridian to send energy down the body. It can be useful in the first trimester if the Stomach is failing to anchor the Penetrating Vessel energy, leading to nausea and feelings of energy rising up the body. This point will help energy to move down the body.

Lung 7 (LU-7)   This is above the styloid process of the radius, 1.5 thumbwidths above the transverse crease of the wrist (Fig. 7.11). Open the mother's thumb and index finger, and slide her other hand in the space between them. The index finger should meet the point on the wrist.

This point is an important point to clear the chest, as well as the head and neck. It is a key point for regulating the Conception Vessel and is used for regulating the flow of Ki to the Uterus and therefore for nourishing the baby in the womb.

Triple Heater   This is easiest to work with the mother sitting or supine. Place her hand on her opposite shoulder so that her arm is bent across her body. The Triple Heater is the meridian on the outside of the arm. You can palm or use your thumbs. There are some important points around the wrist between the radius and ulnar (Fig. 7.12):

- TH-3 – on the dorsum of the hand, just in from the fourth and fifth joints
- TH-4 – is on the wrist

- TH-5 – 2 cun up the arm away from the wrist
- TH-6 – 3 cun up the arm away from the wrist.

Why? The Triple Heater helps to move fluids so it is useful for oedema. The points on the wrist are useful for carpal tunnel syndrome. The Triple Heater strengthens the immune system and helps to integrate changes, both emotional and those to do with temperature.

Lymph pump and lymphatic stroking For this you have two choices:

1. With the mother's arm extended and resting against your body, holding her hand at her wrist, move your hips up and down so that you are pumping the arm but keeping your hands and wrist relaxed (Fig. 7.13A).
2. With the mother's arm bent and supported at the elbow, move your hips up and down to pump the arm (Fig. 7.13B).

It is often suggested that lymph responds to work in groups of five. So you can pump the arm five times, rest and then pump again.

Lymphatic stroking After the lymph pump, you can stroke along the Lung, Heart Protector and Triple Heater. Use feather-light and very slow (as slow as you can and slower than you think) strokes in one direction only from the elbow to the axilla for a few minutes until the puffiness reduces (Fig. 7.14). Afterwards, work from the wrist to the elbow. Finish with some gentle rotations of the hand. It is important to work in this sequence so that the lymphatic system is supported rather than overloaded. The mother will need to drink water immediately afterwards and ensure that she drinks frequently in the next 24 h to help her process any toxins which may be released.

Why? With the arm elevated, you are enabling lymph to flow back and therefore it helps with easing oedema. The lymph pump stimulates the axillary lymph nodes and the light stroking in between the major lymph nodes to the axilla helps to encourage the flow and uptake of lymph. Both techniques are helpful in cases of oedema, often linked with carpal tunnel syndrome, in the

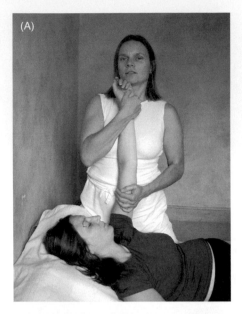

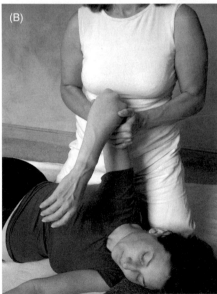

Figure 7.13 A and B: Working the lymph pump in the two positions. Note the practitioner's body – movement comes from the hara moving up and down, so that the practitioner's shoulders and arms can remain relaxed and do not pull on the mother's arm.

arm or poor circulation. They are useful techniques postnatally for inflammation in the breasts or blocked milk ducts.

Caution This type of work should only be done if the oedema is not related to heart or kidney

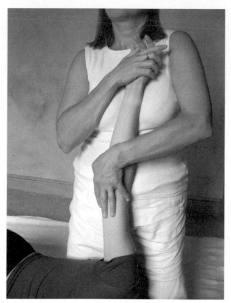

Figure 7.14   Lymphatic stroking.

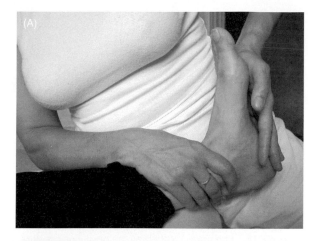

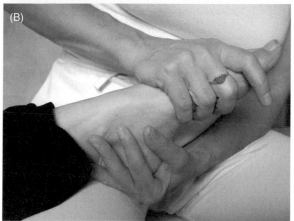

Figure 7.15   A and B: Leg/foot stretch.

failure, as in, for example, pre-eclampsia, as it would place extra burdens on an already compromised system. This kind of oedema would be hard and pit on touch. Oedema which feels puffy and fluidy is caused by Ki not flowing and therefore responds well to this type of work. It is not recommended in the first trimester when there are many changes in fluid and energy flow and the focus is on allowing energy to settle in the uterus.

Legs

In pregnancy, there is often congestion in the legs because of the weight of the baby 'blocking' energy flowing down to them, as well as the increased blood flow. This relates to the energy of the Yin meridians of the legs – Spleen, Liver and Kidney. Oedema in the legs and varicose veins is mainly related to Spleen energy not flowing (this governs transportation and transformation of fluids as well as keeping the blood in the blood vessels) as well as the energy of the Kidney and Bladder (which regulate fluids).

In Chapter 6, we covered many points in the legs, as well as how to work the Bladder meridian. This can be worked easily with the mother lying on her side.

Leg and foot stretches

For these, the mother either needs to be lying or sitting. Sit at the mother's feet with your hara facing the outside of her foot. Place one hand on the back of her ankle and the other on the sole of her foot (Fig. 7.15A). Relax your shoulders and lean your body towards the mother's head. This will stretch the back of her leg and the Bladder meridian. Lean away from her head and this will stretch the front of her leg and the Stomach meridian (Fig. 7.15B). You can repeat this a few times. When you have finished, hold the foot and apply pressure with both hands.

Why?   Stretches work more dynamically: palming or working down the Bladder meridian is beneficial in pregnancy. It is useful for leg

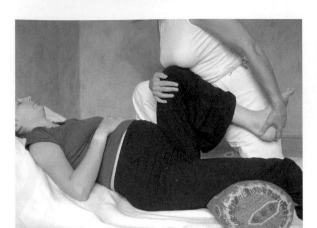

Figure 7.16   Leg pump. Note how the practitioner's hara supports the leg so that it is no effort to move their body in and out, and therefore move the leg.

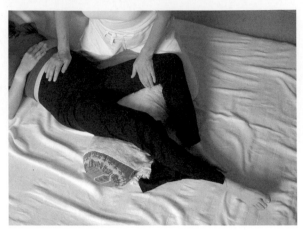

Figure 7.17   Working the Spleen meridian in the leg. Note how the hara of the practitioner is between her two hands.

cramps, pain/tightness in the ankle and calves, balancing fluids such as in cases of oedema and urinary problems, calming and support (both physical and emotional). Refer back to page 110 for information on specific points. You simply need to adapt your position to whatever position the mother is in.

For information on Stomach see page 133.

Yin meridians in the legs

Leg pump   This has the same effect for the inguinal lymph nodes as the arm lymph pump. Gently hold the knee, and pump the leg in and out towards the mother's abdomen as far as it will comfortably go (Fig. 7.16). If it feels comfortable, especially for her back, you can gently circle the leg. Make sure that your hara is behind the knee so your body and shoulders are relaxed.

Spleen meridian   With the mother on her back, place her leg nearest you with the toes resting against the heel of the other leg (Fig. 7.17). Let the mother's knee open out as much as is comfortable for her and then support her leg in this position, either with cushions or your own body. This opens the Spleen meridian. You can have your mother hand on the hara, and with your other hand palm from the foot up the meridian. You can follow this up with thumb pressures. The Spleen is against the tibia. If there is oedema, you can stroke the Spleen meridian in the same way as we did the lymphatic stroking in the arms

i.e. medially to distally, from the knee to the groin and then from the ankle to the knee. The same cautions regarding oedema should be applied as with the arm pump, and the leg should not be lymphatically stroked in the first trimester as this directly affects energy flow to the uterus and may interfere with the delicate balance of energies.

Spleen 4 (SP-4)   Find SP-3 which is on the medial side of the foot in the depression proximal and inferior to the head of the first metatarsal bone. Slide along until you find the next depression. This is SP-4, an important point for nourishing the Blood and the Penetrating Vessel.

Why?   In the first trimester, the Spleen helps to hold the energy of the developing embryo in the uterus by allowing energy to flow up to it and holding this energy in. Weak Spleen energy is sometimes a cause of miscarriage. Later on, working with the Spleen can help with tiredness, especially muscular tiredness related to 'dragging down' feelings in the lower abdomen and heavy legs. It is useful for varicose veins and oedema in the legs, and supports the processes of digestion. Emotionally, it allows the mother to feel more grounded and connected with her body and the baby.

Caution   Avoid using strong pressure over SP-6 as this can over-stimulate the uterus (see page 113).

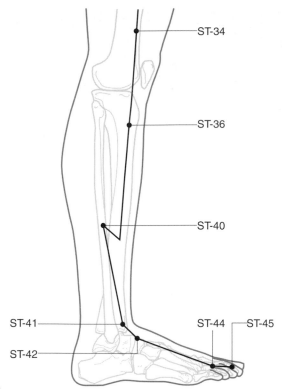

Figure 7.18   The Stomach meridian in the leg with ST-34, ST-36 and ST-40.

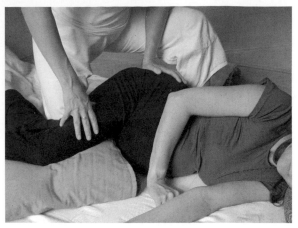

Figure 7.19   Working the Gall Bladder meridian in the side position.

Holding, energetic connections are fine. Don't work the leg if you suspect the mother has deep vein thrombosis (DVT). If the mother has varicose veins, don't work directly over them.

Yang meridians in the legs

Stomach meridian   To work the Stomach, the leg needs to be extended. The Stomach is the main meridian at the front of the leg. Use your mother hand on the mother's hara and use pressure with the working hand from the top down.

ST-34 is in the depression 2 cun above the supero-lateral border of the patella (Fig. 7.18). ST-36 has already been covered in Chapter 6 (p. 112). ST-40 is 8 cun below the knee, one finger breadth lateral to the anterior crest of the tibia (Fig. 7.18).

Why?   Working the Stomach can help draw energy down and is especially useful if the mother seems to live in her head and feel disconnected from the rest of her body. In the first trimester, never just do Stomach work without

also doing some work on the Spleen as it could tend to draw energy away from the uterus, although it can be very useful when combined with other work for nausea. Once the pregnancy is established and stable, it can help with heartburn and ground the mother.

Gall Bladder work   This is easiest to work with the mother in the side position, with the leg further away from the floor bent in front of her at 90°. In this position, Gall Bladder is the meridian on the outside of the leg.

Have the mother hand in the centre of the buttock and work with palm pressure, followed by thumb pressures, along the side of the leg (Fig. 7.19). You can palm over GB-34 (p. 112) but don't over-stimulate it as one of its actions is to help to dilate the cervix.

Other important points and point combinations

Kidney   KI-3 is midway between the tip of the medial malleolus and the tendo calcaneus, i.e. inside one half the distance between the Achilles tendon and the tip of the ankle bone (Fig. 7.20).

KI-6 is in the depression 0.5 cun directly below the inferior border of the medial malleolus.

KI-7 is 2 cun above KI-3, on the anterior border of the tendo calcaneus.

Why?   Kidney is a key energy in pregnancy as it stores Essence which needs to circulate to the baby.

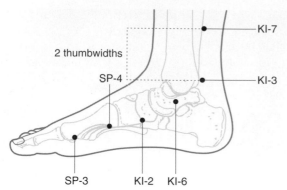

Figure 7.20 Points of the foot with the Kidney points KI-2, KI-3, KI-6, KI-7, SP-3 and SP-4.

Point combinations

The most important point combinations in pregnancy are those which balance the energy of the extraordinary vessels. By holding the relevant two points, the energy of the extraordinary vessel is activated; it is a powerful yet simple way of balancing the energy of these vessels. You hold the two points and feel which is the most Kyo and Jitsu, and then stay holding them until you feel a shift and an evening out of the energy between the two. Sometimes this can happen after a few seconds, sometimes it can take a few minutes. This can be done in labour and postnatally for both mother and baby. You can either hold the two points on the same side and then reverse sides or hold two points on different sides and then reverse.

Penetrating Vessel (SP-4 and HP-6), Conception Vessel (L-7 and K-6), Governing Vessel (SI-3 and BL-62)

SI-3 is on the outside border of the hand, in the depression below the head of the fifth metcarpal bone (Fig. 7.21). BL-62 is 0.5 cun below the lower border of the outside ankle bone (Fig. 6.28 on p. 110).

Girdle Vessel (TH-5 and GB-41)

GB-41 is in the depression between the fourth and fifth metatarsal bones, on the lateral side of the tendon which goes to the little toe (Fig. 6.36 on p. 118).

Why? The extraordinary vessels are the force behind all of the changes in the maternity period for both mother and baby, and balancing them can help regulation of most situations.

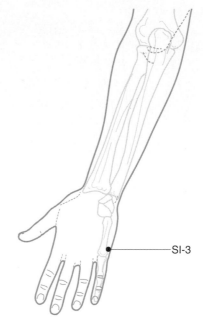

Figure 7.21 Hand point SI-3.

The Penetrating Vessel is especially good for the Blood energy. It may help with conditions such as anaemia, blood flow (especially to nourish the baby but also with varicose veins or bleeding). For nausea/hyperemesis, using the point combination is more effective than just working HP-6 on its own.

The Conception Vessel is especially good for digestion and respiration, while the Governing Vessel is good for the back and low energy. The Girdle Vessel is good for the pelvis, especially sacro-iliac or symphysis pubis problems, and supporting the deep abdominal muscles.

Case study 7.3   Shiatsu for morning sickness – a community midwife

I treated a mother who was pregnant for the third time and who suffered sickness all the way through her second pregnancy and has had debilitating sickness again.

When I performed the treatment B said that she could not describe how she felt because she couldn't put it into words, but she was very relaxed and felt that it had been very beneficial. I included a full antenatal relaxing shiatsu treatment and worked specifically on HP-6, SP-4 and ST-36 points to help relieve the nausea that B was suffering. B felt that she had been very sensitive to these points as she had more sensation when I was working on these. I could tell that this treatment was effective after about 15 min because of B's breathing. She had drifted into a calm state. At the end of the treatment, which lasted about 45 min to an hour, it was good to see how different B felt and that this could be achieved totally non-invasively and in a form that was obviously very acceptable to B. I advised B that she could continue to work the specific points for sickness and nausea herself or ask her husband to do so.

The postnatal period – mother

As the body has undergone sudden and dramatic changes during labour, the main priority for the mother postnatally is to gently allow her energy to adjust. The pattern is for the energy of the hara to be empty and the energy of the breasts and upper body to be full. In the first few days, to touch, the hara will feel quite full and buzzy, even hot – all qualities you might associate with Jitsu. However, this full energy relates to the changes that the hara/abdomen and its internal organs are still undergoing in the early days. The underlying energy pattern is of a lack of energy. There may be heat – but this is because there is not enough water or Yin energy. We do not want to move this energy away. If we started to do sedation/dispersing techniques on the hara, we would probably come into contact with the Kyo areas underneath. The Kyo areas become more obvious once the uterus has finished contracting.

The postnatal period is potentially one of the most difficult times to work with a woman as her energy is depleted and open to being over-stimulated – especially if she has had a traumatic birth. It is important to focus on techniques which nourish the Kyo (the hara/abdomen) and not only those which focus on the Jitsu (neck, shoulders and breast). An experienced shiatsu practitioner would need to draw on their understanding of all the meridians and may work differently from a midwife trained in shiatsu skills, although the techniques I describe here are often part of the work. This level of understanding requires experience of doing shiatsu – and I would only suggest the midwives who have received some direct training in shiatsu work use shiatsu in the first few weeks postnatally. All postnatal techniques fall under the category of complex techniques.

It is beneficial to work in the first few days, even with women who have had Caesareans, but with gentle, holding techniques – focusing on bringing energy to the hara. All the slower abdominal work is excellent – the abdominal holding, Kidney–Uterus, slow stroking of the Girdle Vessel, gentle palming down the Conception Vessel, holding some of the Conception Vessel points and especially connecting with the lower part of the Governing and Conception Vessel pathways in the perineum. You can apply any of the more gentle techniques with meridians, where relevant. Do get good feedback from the mother about what feels helpful and, if you are unsure, consult an experienced shiatsu practitioner.

Case study 7.4   Urinary retention – a hospital midwife

D was suffering from urinary retention following rotational forceps delivery – the previous evening she was unable to pass more than 50 ml. She had no sensation of needing to pass urine or when urinating. **Managed 450 ml and discussion on ward round resulted in request for residual urine volumes** and if less than 100 ml, a urinary catheter was to be reinserted. I offered to try shiatsu before D was next due to pass urine.

I returned for a 15 min treatment and worked the sacral grooves and Bladder meridian in the back with palming and holding. I left the ward and returned to find D had passed 400 ml urine and had <100 ml residual urine, so thankfully a catheter wasn't needed. The midwives had been concerned that the residual volumes would be greater as D had been drinking jugs of water to try to help and had passed very little urine overnight. However, it looked as though the situation was improving spontaneously and D was beginning to get some sensations back. I went back to the ward several hours later and things continued to improve. D was passing better volumes of urine and her sensation of needing to pass urine was improving. I repeated the shiatsu treatment as before. Over the next couple of days the situation improved and D was discharged home, though it took her several days to resolve completely.

The treatment plan was effective even though I only had two short shiatsu sessions with D. Ideally, I would have liked to have tried two to three sessions per day in the first few days to try to improve the situation quicker. D was feeling very despondent due to her lack of sensation when passing urine so the shiatsu helped improve her self-esteem. I think it would have been helpful to continue shiatsu over the next few weeks as bladder problems can take some time to resolve completely.

Abdomen

Remembering the principle of Kyo and Jitsu, we must first work on the hara before we work on the breasts as the hara will tend to be Kyo in relation to the breasts.

Japanese women would traditionally continue to wear their girdle for about 1 month postnatally.

Breast work

This work can be done either through the clothes or directly on the skin. It is really about what feels comfortable both for you and the mother. In our culture, breasts are much more associated with sexuality than feeding a baby. This is possibly one of the influencing factors on why so many women have breastfeeding problems. In fact, when you work on the breasts, the mother usually finds it relaxing and not threatening at all. The lymphatic pump (p. 130) is a good technique to combine with breast work as it will help clear blockages from the breasts as well as the arms. The main meridians which affect the breasts are the Stomach and Penetrating Vessel (Fig. 7.22). Together they regulate

the quality of the milk. Work with these is important if the mother is having problems with producing enough milk or milk of good quality. If the mother has decided not to breastfeed, then work with the Penetrating Vessel to help it process the need not to produce milk will be helpful. The Penetrating Vessel work shown in the pregnancy section is relevant here (p. 124). If the mother is feeding, it is good to work the Penetrating Vessel in the direction towards the breasts, and if the mother is not feeding then work away from the breasts. Work on the Stomach in the legs (p. 133), especially Stomach 36, is helpful.

Case study 7.5   Postnatal breastfeeding and depression – a community midwife

P, who had just given birth to her second child, had developed puerperal psychosis following her first child. P was very anxious about her postnatal recovery and was receiving prophylactic treatment and counselling support from the community psychiatric services.

On day 2 following the birth (a normal delivery in water, as with her first baby) she began to become anxious about her breastfeeding. All seemed fine and she was given advice and reassurance. Later that evening, I received a phone call from her saying that she could not get her baby to feed properly from her right breast and she was becoming very agitated.

Aware of her previous history, I felt that she required a home visit to reassure her and to try to resolve the problem before night-time. P relied on her husband to care for the baby as she was drowsy owing to the medication she had been prescribed by the psychiatrist.

On examination, her right breast had become very engorged. As she was so agitated I suggested a shiatsu treatment to help her relax. Initially she sat upright and I worked the GV and BL points around the occiput, moving onto palming the GB meridian along the sides of her head and included GV-20 which lifts the mood.

I then worked GB-21 which I hoped would encourage the let-down reflex and moved onto her trunk and worked with Kidney–Uterus and Heart–Uterus energy. I finished by using sweeping strokes along her back. This lady was very responsive to the treatment and her milk began to drop quite rapidly after work to the GB-21 point. Following the treatment, she was dramatically improved in her state of agitation. As she was so calm and her breast was much softer, the baby was able to achieve an effective feed. I felt that this treatment was very effective and was surprised at how dramatically the let-down of milk occurred. P continued to breastfeed without any further serious problems.

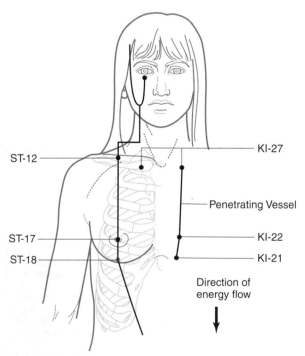

Figure 7.22 The meridians of the breasts – Stomach and Penetrating Vessel with points ST-12, ST-17 and ST-18.

ST-12

ST-17

ST-18

KI-27

Penetrating Vessel

KI-22

KI-21

Direction of energy flow

Stomach torso

The Stomach meridian on the chest flows in a line which passes directly through the nipples. In the abdomen its points lie 2 thumbwidths from the Conception Vessel. The same technique can be used as for the Penetrating Vessel and Conception Vessel in pregnancy (p. 124) – either palming or thumb pressures but this time working towards the breasts. If you are using the thumbs, which are more specific, then you can work both sides at the same time. In this case, you need to use the rest of your hand as the mother hand, cupping it on the side of the mother's body to support the thumb. Make sure that the pressure of the thumb is at 90° into the body. You can do this either through the clothes or directly on the skin (Fig. 7.23).

Why? The Stomach is the main meridian responsible for transforming food energy via blood into breast milk. It is very good for improving the quality of the breast milk, as well as boosting its supply. It also has a strong effect on bringing energy down the body.

Direct shiatsu of the breasts

Using the same kind of thumb technique as we did to work the Stomach, we can use our thumbs all around and indeed over the breasts. Feel for Kyo and Jitsu areas and balance between the two.

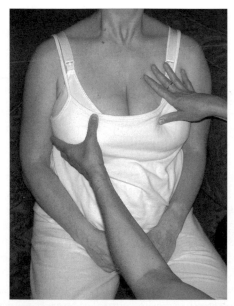

Figure 7.23 Working the Stomach meridian in the breasts for the postnatal mother.

> **Case study 7.6** A reluctant feeder after Caesarean – an independent midwife
>
> Postnatally, the baby was very reluctant to suck at the breasts (which often happens with babies who have had medical analgesia) and the mother found it uncomfortable to sit up for long periods to feed the baby. As the baby was not stimulating the breasts, the production of milk was low. ST-18 and L-1 points were worked on to aid lactation. In 24 h her breasts were starting to fill with milk. The baby was also getting better at latching on to the breasts.
>
> A day later, her breasts were slightly engorged. GB-21, ST-36 and SP-6 were worked to help the flow of milk.

Why? This will help to stimulate the lactate glands, relieve glandular inflammations and help with both the flow and quality of the milk.

Back

Energy is often Jitsu in the upper back and Kyo in the lower back. Use the back techniques to release these Kyo and Jitsu areas. This work will also help to ease breast congestion as well as ease backaches.

Neck and shoulders

The tightness of energy in the breasts is often linked with, or is the cause of, tightness in the neck and shoulders. All the work previously shown is of value, especially Gall Bladder work as it is the Gall Bladder that is responsible for the let-down reflex and for moving energy in the breasts. Gall Bladder work is indicated when milk is not flowing, as opposed to Stomach which is indicated when there are problems with the quality and quantity of milk. GB-21 is a particularly important point for stimulating the let-down reflex.

Arms

Emotionally and physically, it is the energy of fire that predominates in the postnatal period. The loss of Blood during labour means that the fire energy tends to be scattered, and the forming of a new relationship with her baby draws upon fire. It is useful to work the Heart Protector in the arms which will support the function of the Heart. Remember HP-8 is an important point for calming.

Work on the Stomach will help to balance this as earth provides the basis for anchoring fire energy.

Case study 7.7   Breastfeeding mum – a hospital midwife and midwife shiatsu practitioner

J had a 13-week-old baby delivered at 35 weeks following induced labour for premature rupture of the membranes. Baby J was admitted to the neonatal unit with birth asphyxia but recovered well. J was feeling quite stressed as she had already returned to part-time work and was still traumatized by her experience of baby J's birth; she was also very anxious about her milk supply. Baby J was feeding frequently but not very well from one breast in particular.

Treatment 1
This was neck and head for general stress relief, followed by hara massage and palming to ST-36, the Heart–Uterus connection to help balance emotions continuing up CV to K-27 including some of the breast points. The treatment finished by holding SP-4 and HP-6 to balance PV to help the milk supply.

Feedback
J had a dramatic improvement in her milk supply. Baby J was settling and sleeping for 4 h between feeds although still reluctant to feed on one side. J also felt more energetic and was sleeping better too.

Treatment 2
J was still quite stressed and baby J had just been discharged from hospital following chest problems. Feeding was still difficult on one side, but lactation was generally better. Shiatsu in the side position was given to access neck and shoulders better. The treatment focused on neck points, shoulder blades, back, arms including 'lymph pump' to really get lactation going. It continued down the legs following the GB meridians SP-4 and HP-6 to finish and boost milk supply. Heart–Uterus to the front of the body.

Feedback
Lactation continued to improve. Baby J was taking to both sides and feeding well. The mother was also sleeping better, with more energy. The baby was massaged and Lung Shu (*this is another way of referring to the Lung points on the back on the Bladder meridian*) points were used to help with the chest condition.

J had never had shiatsu before and was very pleased with her response to her treatments. In fact she was quite sceptical about shiatsu but thought she would just see. J is now having regular treatment and is thinking of training in shiatsu herself.

Postnatal care for the baby

We could say that the baby's first experience of 'shiatsu' is from when it is aware of the sense of touch from within the womb. Babies often respond to the mother receiving shiatsu while pregnant. The journey of labour, with its contractions, is like a very vigorous shiatsu for the baby. Simple skin-to-skin holding when the baby is first born can include gently holding some of the specific meridians, especially the Governing Vessel. An experienced shiatsu practitioner may even be able to stimulate specific points to help a baby begin to breathe or to help a baby suffering from breathing difficulties.

For the first few weeks, the work is about encouraging new parents to bond with their baby and for the baby to feel comfortable with being touched with human hands and becoming accustomed to its new environment. This can include techniques that stimulate the relevant meridians. In these early days, a good position to work with babies is with the mother holding them, often against their chest, and having skin-to-skin contact. We work directly on the skin using oils – although oil isn't always necessary in the first few days. It is good to encourage the mum and dad to do massage/shiatsu with their baby daily as part of the routine and to see it as something enjoyable – a special time with their baby – rather than a chore. As a midwife, you could talk the mother and father through some of the following sequences, getting them to work, or you may do a combination of you working on the baby along with them. Depending on how much you are used to working with babies, you may need to do some further baby massage or baby shiatsu training. Some midwives teach baby massage/shiatsu classes for new parents postnatally (see p. 68, Case study 4.7).

We apply the same basic principles when working with babies, respecting the different size and weight of the baby. Pressure is much less and we don't need to move around the body to reach all the different areas and meridians. Babies' energy is very Yang because they are in a stage of intense growth and outward movement of energy, and their bodies have not built up imbalances in energy flow which have become held deeply in the body; their energy thus responds quickly and easily. Work with babies means holding for shorter amounts of time and involves more stroking movements, rather than lots of holding, unless they have suffered from trauma, when holding work is beneficial.

As babies are developing their bodies, we need to be able to respond to the different movements that they make. They present to us the meridians they want to be worked on. As the baby passes through the different developmental stages, such as being able to lift the head in prone, sit, crawl and eventually walk, we find that our work changes. Initially, we will work more with the baby in supine or prone positions, but later on sitting or side will be good to work with. Working with babies means responding to their different needs and respecting how long they want to be worked. Like with all shiatsu, it is hard to give a time. For one baby 5 min may be too long and for another, half an hour not long enough. An average time is probably about 15–20 min, but this can vary enormously from day to day. As with all shiatsu, be guided by the baby's response. If they are getting tired, restless or simply not enjoying being touched anymore, then the parents need to stop and cuddle them.

However, don't be afraid of working with a crying baby. Sometimes crying can indicate a release of trauma and shiatsu may help the baby process that trauma – usually related to the birth and more common in instrumentally delivered babies. This type of crying is different from a pure cry of distress – it feels like the baby is processing something and the cry lessens in intensity if the shiatsu is helping. Detailed descriptions of work with babies who have suffered trauma are outside the scope of this book, but it is always worth trying to gradually encourage the baby to enjoy touch. If the baby is crying, often very gentle holding work is what is needed – sometimes even holding off the body. Many people avoid touching babies who cry when touched – but sensitive work may help the baby process the trauma. Not working at all often means that the patterns of pain which could have been quite easily released become more deeply held in the body. There is increasing evidence of how unprocessed birth trauma can stay in the body for the rest of our lives (Castellino, unpublished work, 1996, Chamberlain 1988, Emerson, unpublished work, 1996, Janov 1983, Noble 1993, Verny 1992).

Ideally, in one session, we would aim to cover all the meridians to ensure an even flow of energy, even if this is simply a gentle stroking over all areas. This means having the baby in both the prone and supine positions. With today's guidance on 'back to sleep' many parents never put their babies on their fronts and this is an important part of their development. If there is less time, then focus on the more Kyo areas initially which will be the areas that the baby likes. Gradually focus on the more Jitsu areas, encouraging the baby to feel more comfortable with them.

Stretches and movements

Working with babies is very much about observing the movements they do and encouraging them to develop and expand them. This way you help to promote even development of the meridians. It is important to see this as working with the baby, rather than forcing them to do something. Any movement should feel like the baby relaxes into a larger movement, rather than being forced into it. If the baby always objects to a particular movement, this can indicate a problem, either physically or energetically, and it is worth seeking further advice either from a shiatsu practitioner, the baby's GP/paediatrician or both.

Oil

With a baby a few day's old, you can either work through the clothes or use oil directly on the skin. If the baby's skin is quite dry, then oil may be helpful. Begin by warming the oil in your hands and then lightly stroke the oil over the baby's body. Avoid putting oil on the baby's hands, especially as the baby gets older, so that they don't eat it (although a small amount will probably be fine). Don't put oil on the baby's face as the strokes on the face are light and you want to avoid getting oil in the eyes and mouth. Oil can be applied to the baby's head, depending on how much hair the baby has. If the baby has a lot of hair, it is best not to use too much oil as it will make the hair greasy. If the baby has little hair, then oil will be fine to use.

Hara

This area is open with a baby and they may be calmed easily as you hold it. If there is trauma held here then the baby may initially respond by being unsettled and you may need to hold the

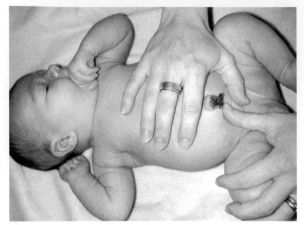

Figure 7.24 A mother working on a newborn baby's hara – holding the Kyo and Jitsu areas with the fingertips.

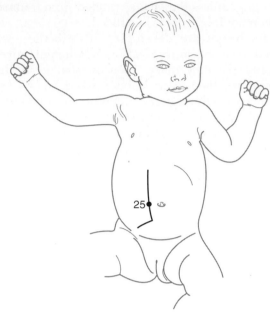

Figure 7.25 Stomach 25.

baby away from your body with an energetic focus, gradually getting them comfortable with physical touch. In the first few days, with the healing of the umbilical cord, you want to avoid direct physical stimulation over and around the umbilicus. Holding lightly around the area, and connecting more energetically, is beneficial.

Working with the hara will help balance all of the baby's energy as it includes diagnostic areas for the whole body. As the digestive organs are in the hara area, then work here is especially useful for any kind of digestive problem – wind, colic and constipation.

Techniques Place one hand on the baby's hara and the other under their back. Feel the baby's breathing through your hands. After a while, move the hand on the front very lightly round in a clockwise direction – you may find that using the whole palm of the hand is clumsy and use the tips of the fingers instead. As you do this, feel which areas are more Kyo and which are more Jitsu. If you are getting parents to feel this, just get them to feel 'hard' and 'soft' areas. Balance Kyo and Jitsu as with any other area. Hold the Kyo areas first with a soft part of the hand and allow the area to warm and fill. This happens much more quickly and with much less pressure than with adults. Afterwards hold the Jitsu areas a little more firmly with the aim of moving tightness away. You can finish by holding the Kyo and Jitsu areas at the same time until you feel they are fairly balanced and then palming around the abdomen (Fig. 7.24).

Stomach 25

This is 2 cun (i.e. baby thumbwidths) to each side of the navel (Fig. 7.25). This is the Large Intestine Bo point which means that it balances the organ of the Large Intestine. It is especially useful for constipation or diarrhoea. To work it, hold the point with one thumb, while the other hand supports the back. Feel how hard or soft it is. If it is hard, work with a slow, circular movement until the hardness eases. If it is soft, hold until you feel it filling up. The response can sometimes be quite immediate, so be ready with a nappy!

Legs

The legs can be very calming for the baby. They relate more to the physical energy, and the arms to the emotional energy of a person. Specific meridians we would want to focus on are the Stomach and Spleen as they are earth meridians. They help the baby make the adjustment to being in the world and relating to the mother in a different way. They also relate to the digestion and intake of food.

Techniques We can use the hand-over-hand stroking movement down the baby's legs to the

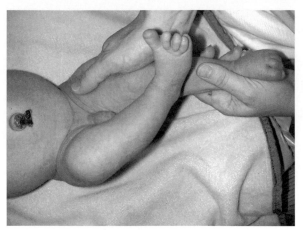

Figure 7.26   Working the Stomach on a baby's legs.

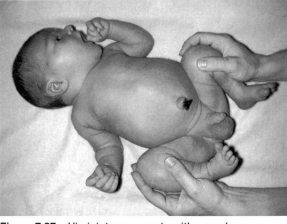

Figure 7.27   Hip joint movements with a newborn.

foot (Fig. 7.26). This can be varied so it can be very light or firmer, slow or quicker. If the baby doesn't like the stroking, then they may prefer a firmer touch – you can gently grasp down the legs. As the baby gets older, the pressure will get firmer (especially as the baby begins to flesh out in the legs) then kneading-type techniques can be beneficial and fun.

These types of techniques can be focused on the meridians. Stomach is the main meridian on the front of the leg – you can stroke or knead down this to follow the traditional flow of energy. Spleen is the most important on the inside of the leg – you can focus your movements on moving from foot to groin.

Stomach 36 (ST-36)

This is an important point on babies for balancing Ki flow. It can be both emotionally and physically settling.

Leg/hip movements

Even a young baby may enjoy gentle hip rotations, similar to the hip joint test, but without the pressure. It is best to do these with no nappy on the baby, as this allows greater freedom of movement.

Bring the baby's knees into their tummy as much as they will let you (Fig. 7.27). Gently open out the hips, like in the hip joint test. If the baby resists don't go further. Then gently extend the baby's legs.

Why?   This works all the meridians of the legs and hips, and promotes their energy flow and development. Often a baby will prefer one part of the movement, and this movement encourages them to be more comfortable with all parts and therefore relate to all the meridians.

Feet

As the main beginning and ending points for the meridians are in the feet, work on them influences the whole meridian.

General holding and stroking on the feet is usually quite soothing for the baby and can often help with digestive problems because, by working with the feet, you are effectively influencing energy flow in the whole body.

Techniques   Stroke over the top of the foot and on the bottom of the foot – not too lightly otherwise the baby will find it ticklish.

It is good to gently pull out each toe. You can use a slight rolling movement if the baby prefers this. Pause when you reach the base of each nail – this is where many of the points are – and gently apply a little pressure. You can also try to stroke in between the toes.

You can stroke the feet against each other and even gently tap them together.

As the baby gets bigger, it will become fascinated with its feet and you can play all sorts of fun movement and clapping games – singing things like 'this little piggy went to market'.

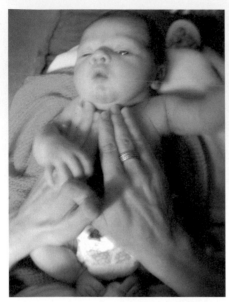

Figure 7.28   Working on the newborn baby's chest.

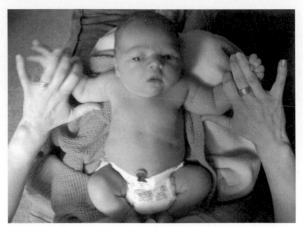

Figure 7.29   Opening the baby's arms and holding HP-6 and HP-8.

Chest

The chest is quite important as it has the main pathways of the Penetrating and Conception Vessels flowing through it. As the baby is going through a period of great change and adaptation, these meridians are important for regulating overall energy. As the baby gradually uncurls from the fetal position, then the Yin meridians of the front come to the front. Don't force this opening movement, but working these meridians will help to support it. The chest is also important because the baby is adapting to breathing as well as being susceptible to its environment and will often suffer from slight congestion in this area.

Techniques   With the hands on the abdomen, you can gently stroke up the midline (covering CV and PV) (Fig. 7.28) and then out over to under the clavicles (Lung area), and stroke down the side of the body (the main meridian here is the GB).

An alternative is to use gentle pressures – keep one hand on the hara and with the other use either your thumb pad, or the side of the hand or fingertips to apply gentle pressure either up or down the midline. Pressure can be applied to LU-1 and LU-2.

Arms

These tend to relate more to the emotions. Often newborn babies will not like their arms being worked – especially if you try to open them up to expose the Yin meridians. They have been used to being curled up in the fetal position, protected, and need to take their time to open up to the world. It is important to respect this and gently encourage them to open up. The Heart Protector is the most important Yin meridian in the arms for the baby – in the womb, the mother acted to fulfil the baby's Heart Protector function. Opposite the Heart Protector, on the outside of the arms, is the Triple Heater, which helps to regulate body temperature and the immune system.

Techniques   From the chest, stroke out over the arms, focusing on encouraging the inside to open up (Fig. 7.29). If the baby doesn't like this, then gently stroke the arms in whichever position the baby is most comfortable.

You can also try gentle pressures – your fingers may be enough.

If the baby is happy to open out its arms, then you can slowly open and close.

Gentle pressures or stroking along the middle of the inside of the arm (Heart Protector) are calming. You can hold HP-6. You can also stroke along the outside of the arm.

Hand

You can play with this, like the foot, using pressures and stroking on the front and back of the hand and gently opening each finger. HP-8, right in the middle of the palm of the hand, is very calming.

Head and neck

Often this is where birth trauma is stored, especially if the head was stuck, or the baby was delivered by forceps or ventouse. If this was the case, the baby is usually extremely sensitive to having the head touched, even lightly, but encouraging the baby to feel happy with touch will help it process the trauma.

Caesarean babies who have not had the same moulding and compression to the head as with vaginally delivered babies will benefit from gentle compression techniques and usually enjoy them. The main meridian of the head to focus on is the Governing Vessel.

Techniques   It is good to have the baby close to you, and a good time for the mum to work on the baby's head is while it is feeding. Another position is to have the baby's head cradled in the mother's lap, feet away from the mother.

Cradling head   Lightly place one or both hands on either side of the skull, making contact with the heel, palm and fingers in a cupping action. If the baby is happy with light pressure, increase the pressure slightly until you are holding the head as firmly as feels comfortable for the baby. You may find that the baby likes more pressure with one part of your hand only. Feel if one side of the head is more Kyo or Jitsu. Allow energy to flow between your two hands.

You can keep the palms still and do some gentle stroking movements with your fingers, as though you are rubbing shampoo into the baby's head.

CV/GV   Begin by placing one thumb on top of the other over the area between the baby's eyebrows, while you keep the rest of your hand cupped around the baby's head (Fig. 7.30). Feel if this area is Kyo or Jitsu and respond accordingly. From here, use your thumbs to work up the midline to GV-20 just in front of the crown of the head. As you go over the fontanelles, be careful not to apply too much pressure. When you reach GV-20, you may be able to apply a little firmer pressure here. You can then work down the back of the

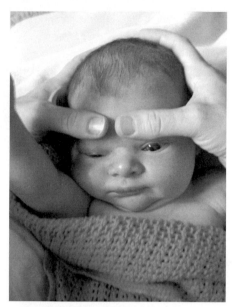

Figure 7.30   Working a newborn baby's head.

head till GV-15 between BL-20. You can finish by cradling the base of the skull in your fingers.

This kind of work is very helpful if the baby's head is very bruised, swollen or asymmetrical, either from an instrumental delivery or just a long, hard birth. Work will need to be done very sensitively, but if you work to balance the Kyo and Jitsu areas on the head, energy changes very easily.

Why?   The Governing Vessel and Conception Vessel are the main meridians that would be affected by any birth trauma, and work with these can balance energy quite profoundly. The baby may cry, but if the cry gradually lessens in intensity then continue working gently.

Face

There are many important points on the face (Fig. 7.31). One important pathway is the Bladder meridian which starts at the inside of the eye. The other is the Stomach which goes from the centre of the eye down in a straight line to the edge of the mouth. LI-20 is at the base of each nostril and helps to clear the nose.

Technique   To work the face, cup the head in your hands and gently place your thumbs on top of each other over the point/meridian that you

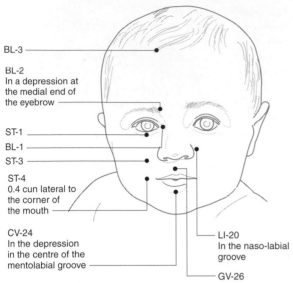

BL-3

BL-2
In a depression at
the medial end of
the eyebrow

ST-1

BL-1

ST-3

ST-4
0.4 cun lateral to
the corner of
the mouth

CV-24
In the depression
in the centre of the
mentolabial groove

LI-20
In the naso-labial
groove

GV-26

Figure 7.31   Meridians and points on the baby's face. The Bladder, Stomach, Governing Vessel and Conception Vessel meridians and BL-1, BL-2, ST-1, LI-20.

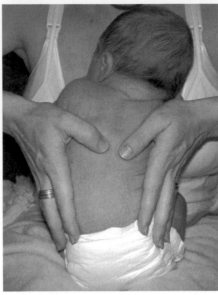

Figure 7.32   Working down a newborn baby's back. Note how the mother can use her body to support the baby.

wish to work. If the thumbs are too heavy, then you can use any of the other fingers. The little finger will be the lightest. Hold the points.

Back

Birth affects the spine which relates to the GV and also the Bladder meridian. Work with the back will balance both the structure and the energy. Holding is often very relaxing.

   Position   The baby can lay face down on the ground, although if it doesn't find this comfortable it can be held against the mother's body or she can sit and rest the baby over her legs.

   Techniques   Hold the base of the skull in the centre, and the centre of the base of the sacrum with your fingertips. See if you can feel energy flowing between the two points along the length of the spine. This may be sufficient.

   You can also gently palm down the spine. You can use light circling movements with your fingertips or thumb down the spine and to each side (Fig. 7.32). You can palm out from each side (BL). Then more massage-type strokes such as kneading can be used.

> **Case study 7.8   Mucousy baby – a hospital midwife**
>
> I treated a mucousy baby who was't keen to fix at the breast for a feed. I sat with the baby lying on my knee and worked the Lung and Heart Protector meridians for a few minutes. He promptly vomited some mucous. I treated LI-20 on the side of the base of the nose.
>
>   He still wasn't very keen to breastfeed; however he had a few sucks at the breast which was at least a start. Unfortunately I was short of time and was unable to return to do further shiatsu. Feeding improved and the baby went home breastfeeding well. It was a short treatment due to lack of time but it still seemed to be effective. Gentle palming down the Heart Protector on the arms appeared to work quickly. Stroking the Governing Vessel and Conception Vessel would have helped the meridians and could have been used in further treatments. Mum was happy for him to have shiatsu as she was obviously anxious that he wasn't keen to feed. Subsequently, she was more relaxed when he began to have a few sucks at the breast. This helped the bonding between mum and baby.

Checklist of specific conditions

This is a checklist aimed at midwives and shiatsu practitioners. For shiatsu practitioners unfamiliar with maternity work, you will need to make sure that you have an understanding of the conditions so that you know when to work alongside a midwife and conventional medical care. For parents, it is important to check what you are intending to do with a midwife, doctor or shiatsu practitioner first. This list isn't necessarily exhaustive, it only includes techniques covered in this book. You need to refer back to the practical sections and also the theory to build up a complete picture of what you may be able to do. Remember that you can also do the relevant meridian exercise (Chapter 8) or visualization (see earlier in this section).

For each condition, I will give some meridian work suggestions – the meridian names will be written out in full and not abbreviated. I will also give some suggestions for specific points – these will be abbreviated to help distinguish them from the meridians.

Note: whenever I give meridian work on the Conception Vessel, Governing Vessel, Penetrating Vessel and Girdle Vessel, please remember to include their point combinations, namely L-7 and KI-6, BL-62 and SI-3, SP-4 and HP-6, and TH-5 and GB-41.

Pregnancy

Abdominal pain

For all pain, work with the general abdominal holding technique. The Conception Vessel brings energy to the centre. The Spleen in the legs brings energy up and supports muscle and organs; the Kidney and Kidney–Uterus support deep energy and help with fatigue; the Penetrating Vessel balances Blood energy; the Heart–Uterus balances Blood energy, is emotionally calming for the baby and helps the mother's connection with the baby. The Girdle Vessel can support ligaments, joints and deep abdominal muscles as well as helping to balance energy from front to back.

Visualization of the baby in the womb will help the mother to connect in a positive way with any pain. CV-3–5 and Uterus points all help with abdominal pain

For superficial achiness as opposed to deep internal pain, use abdominal stroking and holds.

For 'dragging down' heaviness in muscle, the Spleen brings energy up and supports muscle.

For deep internal feelings of pain (possible prolapse of organs), work up the Governing Vessel and Spleen.

For Caesarean scar pain work the Spleen and Kidney.

For ligament pain, especially the uterine round ligaments, work the Spleen/Girdle Vessel, and Gall Bladder in the legs.

For symphysis pubis pain, work CV-2 and the pubic bone.

For heartburn and epigastric pain, work the Stomach, chest and legs, CV-12 (Stomach point) and HP-6.

Amnniotic fluid

Water energy and Essence regulate the conditions of both too much and not enough fluid, i.e. polyhydramnios and oligohydramnios.

They can relate to fear and overprotecting, or not protecting the baby – Bladder, Kidney, Heart Protector and Triple Heater. The Triple Heater also helps to regulate fluids.

BL-23 benefits Kidney.

BL-25 benefits Bladder.

BL-22 benefits Triple Heater.

CV-4 benefits Essence.

Anaemia

You need to work with Blood: Stomach, Spleen, Penetrating Vessel, Heart–Uterus.

Use the Blood visualization.

BL-18 benefits Liver, important for Blood.

BL-23 benefits Kidney.

BL-20 benefits Spleen.

BL-17 benefits Blood.

BL-33 promotes formation of Blood along with BL-20.

BL-52 benefits Kidney and Essence.

CV-4 benefits Kidney and Uterus.

Anxiety

Work with the Bladder for support and to calm feelings of fear; the Penetrating Vessel, Spleen and Stomach to settle the energy down; and the Heart–Uterus and Heart Protector to settle emotions.

CV-4 calms deep fear.

HT-7, HP-8 and KI-1 are all calming.

Baby in womb

Reduced fetal movements Work the Heart–Uterus (to help the mother to connect), Kidney–Uterus (to nourish the baby), Bladder back, including the sacrum, and legs, light holding, but not excessive stimulation, to stimulate flow and movement.

Work BL-67 gently, not so much as when working to turn breech babies, just to get the baby moving.

Mother not connecting or anxiety about baby Work the Heart–Uterus, Heart Protector, CV-4.

Intrauterine growth retardation (IUGR) The baby is not being nourished by Ki, Blood and Essence. Ensure the flow of Essence by working with the Kidney–Uterus, Conception Vessel and KI-1.

Ensure the flow of Blood energy by working with the Spleen, Heart–Uterus (see other Blood points under Anaemia).

Ensure the flow of Ki by working the Conception Vessel and Governing Vessel, and work towards the Uterus and Girdle Vessel using gentle sacral and abdominal work.

ST-36 nourishes Liver Blood.

CV-12 tonifies the Stomach and Spleen to produce Ki and Blood.

Incorrect position See Pre-labour later in this chapter.

Backache – upper, lower, and including neck and shoulders

Remember that the upper and lower back are related. For the lower back you sometimes need to work the upper and vice versa.

Upper and lower backache Work the Governing Vessel, Bladder and Kidney back. Focus on balancing Kyo and Jitsu. Work the Bladder legs.

Upper back Pain here is often caused by wood energy rising so also include work on the neck and shoulders, especially the Gall Bladder, Bladder, Governing Vessel. You may need to work the Lung and Heart Protector on the front to balance (these are often Kyo).

Use the three-point shoulder release and scapula release.

GB-20, BL-10 and GV-20 all release energy in the neck and upper back.

Lower back Work the Kidney–Uterus, as often there is low energy here.

Until about 16 weeks, avoid working the sacrum, apart from gentle holding and connections. Afterwards, use sacral opening or closing techniques and BL-31–34.

BL-23 benefits the Kidneys, and BL-47 and BL-48 help to ease sciatica and lumbosacral pain.

Bleeding, vaginal

This is usually due to the Spleen not holding blood in/up.

Work the Spleen legs. Work upwards on the Conception Vessel and Penetrating Vessel.

GV-20 brings energy up.

ST-36 strengthens Ki.

CV-3–5 and BL-34 all help stop uterine bleeding.

Breathlessness

This is related to the Lungs being affected by the baby drawing on the mother's Kidney energy, and to energy not flowing in the upper burner.

Work the Conception Vessel, Penetrating Vessel, Kidney–Uterus, Kidney back, and Lung including L-1, L-2 and L-7. Work the Heart Protector including HP-6. These all tend to be Kyo. The upper back and shoulders tend to be Jitsu (see above). Use side stretches to open the ribs, and arm movements and stretches to open the Lung.

BL-23 benefits Kidney.

BL-25 benefits Triple Heater which regulates the upper burner.

BL-13 benefits Lung.

KI-1 draws energy down.

Carpal tunnel syndrome

This is either caused by tightness in the neck and shoulders (see the upper back work) or fluids building up in the arm – work the Lung, Heart Protector and Triple Heater, Lymph pump.

HP-6, HP-7 and TH-4, TH-5 and TH-6 all free energy and fluids in the wrist.

Colds, sinus congestion

This is usually due to Bladder and Lung energy not flowing, so work with them. The mother may also have tightness around the neck and shoulders (see backache).

Use gentle pressures and stroking around the sinuses.

GB-20, BL-10, BL-2, ST-3, LI-20 and L1 all help to clear sinuses.

Constipation

This is due to dryness of fluids, and Yin and Ki not flowing. Work with the Spleen and Kidney helps to move fluids. Use abdominal work – especially the Conception Vessel and Girdle Vessel. General work with gentle stretches will help to move energy round the body, but avoid working on 'induction' points.

ST-36 nourishes Ki and Blood, promotes bowel movement.

BL-23 benefits Kidney.

BL-20 benefits Spleen.

Coughs

This is related to congestion of Ki in the chest, usually affecting the Lung, Kidney, Heart Protector; it is similar to 'breathlessness'.

Diabetes

This is related to the Spleen and Penetrating Vessel which together regulate blood sugar levels in the body, and the Stomach which is about the intake of food energy. Work with these meridians.

ST-36 regulates Ki especially related to digestion.

Dizziness

This is usually a result of Liver energy rising or Spleen energy failing to go down.

Work down the Spleen/Liver leg, and include neck and shoulders work (see above).

GB-20 is good for calming the Liver and working with dizziness.

LV-3 brings energy down but you need to work gently in a general holding way, not in an intense way as for induction. Hold the feet and include KI-1 which helps to settle energy.

Fatigue

This is often due to depletion of Ki, Blood or Essence. Work as for 'Baby – IUGR'. ST-36, LV-13, CV-4, TH-3 and GV-20 are all beneficial for these energies in pregnancy.

Haemorrhoids

The Spleen is not holding Blood in the vessels. Work up the Spleen and Governing Vessel to draw Yang energy up. Use the CV/GV point hold to bring energy to the perineum, self massage around the anus with light stimulation of CV-1 and GV-1.

GV-20, BL-57–58 and BL-32 draw energy up.

BL-20 benefits Spleen.

Headaches

For those related to pre-eclampsia/toxaemia (PET) see Pre-eclampsia.

They are often caused by wood energy rising and getting stuck in the neck and shoulders (see above). This can be caused by a weak Bladder, so you need to work this too. You can work with drawing energy away from here and working the feet.

BL-10, GB-20 and GV-20 are local points to help release the stuck energy; KI-1 draws energy to the feet.

Heartburn

This is usually to do with the Stomach. The middle burner is blocked which can also affect the Heart Protector and Conception Vessel on the front and the Governing Vessel on the back.

BL-21and CV-12 benefit Stomach, ST-36 benefits Stomach and draws energy down, HP-6 can help with Stomach. For the back work the TH-7 area to release the middle burner. Work BL-17 to release the diaphragm.

L-1 can help send energy down.

Hypotension/hypertension

This usually affects the Governing Vessel. You can work the meridian and GV-20 either with a focus on sending energy down for hypertension or drawing energy up for hypotension.

Infertility

This is mainly to do with Essence so you need to work on the Conception Vessel, Penetrating Vessel, Governing Vessel, Kidney and Bladder.

Work to warm the lower abdomen/hara, especially the Heart–Uterus, Kidney–Uterus, Girdle Vessel and lower burner.

Use gentle stretches to move Liver energy.

KI-3, BL-23 and BL-52 tonify the Kidneys, BL-52 nourishes the Essence.

CV-4 strengthens the Uterus and benefits the Kidneys.

GV-4, Ming Men, stokes up fire of the Gate of Life.

CV-8 warms Kidneys and Essence.

The extra points Bao Men and Zihu (correspond with ST-28) benefit the Uterus.

BL-34 benefits Kidney and Essence.

Insomnia

Usually fire energy is out of balance. Work the Heart Protector and Heart–Uterus

HP-6 and HP-8 calm fire energy.

Joints, excessive laxity of – especially sacro-iliac

This is often related to the Liver and Gall Bladder not supporting ligaments.

If the joints of the pelvis are over-lax, this is especially linked with the Girdle Vessel. The Spleen supports muscle.

Leg cramps

Poor circulation (i.e. Blood not nourishing the tissues) and a diet of too much Yin food (i.e. sugar, sweet drinks, cold foods) may be the cause.

Use gentle shiatsu along all the Yang meridians especially the Stomach, Gall Bladder and Bladder in the legs. Do some of the Stomach and Bladder leg stretches.

Bladder points in the legs, especially BL-67 and BL-57, all help with spasms.

Work with the foot especially KI-1.

Ligament pain

This is often related to the Liver and Gall Bladder which control the ligaments and tendons. You can also hold locally in the area of pain, balancing Kyo and Jitsu.

Miscarriage, threatened, actual

This is usually due to weakness of the Kidney and Essence; therefore, work on the Kidney, Kidney–Uterus, Conception Vessel, Governing Vessel, Penetrating Vessel and Girdle Vessel. Also work the Spleen to hold Ki in the Uterus. The Heart Protector and Heart–Uterus are good for calming.

ST-28, the door of the uterus, the door of the baby.

When the baby has died and the mother has not miscarried and wants to deliver her baby naturally, using the induction points can help her miscarry.

Nausea/morning sickness

This is mostly due to Stomach energy not moving down, caused by weak Stomach, Conception Vessel, Kidney, Penetrating Vessel or by Liver energy rising up.

Work down these meridians plus the Heart–Uterus and Spleen.

Work the Stomach leg downwards to bring energy down to the lower parts of the body and finish with feet holding.

The HP-6 and SP-4 combination benefits the Penetrating Vessel, the combination works better than just HP-6 on its own.

ST-34 and ST-36 are powerful points for the Stomach and drawing energy down.

BL-21 benefits Stomach.

BL-20 benefits Spleen.

Muscle, poor tone, tightness

This is related to the Spleen function of holding up and muscle tone not working well. Work the Spleen.

In the abdomen, it relates to the Penetrating Vessel, Conception Vessel and Girdle Vessel flows.

Oedema

If the oedema is accompanied by hypertension and proteinuria, it may be linked with PET (see this entry). In this case, don't do any stroking or lymphatic work, as this may stress the heart and kidneys; be extremely vigilant with all other work and check that it is not aggravating the situation. In severe cases, work should only be done in the controlled environment of a hospital.

If the oedema is simply due to excess fluids, then all of the following work is suitable.

Legs   Use mainly the Bladder, Kidney and Spleen.

Arms   Use mainly the Heart Protector, Triple Heater and Lung; the oedema may affect the Bladder and Kidney.

Use elevated positions of the arms and legs to help drain fluids. Use the lymph pump to stimulate inguinal or axillary lymph nodes.

If the oedema is mild, light, slow stroking towards the lymph nodes is helpful.

For both arms and legs, BL-23 tonifies the Kidney Yang. GV-4 strengthens the fire of the Gate of Life. KI-3 tonifies the Kidneys.

For the legs, BL-22 promotes transformation and excretion of fluids in the lower burner. BL-23 benefits the Kidneys, and ST-36 tonifies Ki and resolves oedema.

For the arms BL-18 moves Liver Ki and eliminates stagnation of the middle burner. BL-15 benefits the Heart, BL-16 benefits the Governing Vessel and moves the energy of the upper burner. TH-4–6 are local points for releasing energy and fluids in the wrist.

Postural hypotension

This is to do with Kidney energy and the Governing Vessel/Conception Vessel circuit. Palm up GV and CV to GV-20. Holding KI-1 benefits the Kidney.

Placenta

Any problems with the functioning of the placenta are to do with Ki, Blood and Essence (see the Baby – IUGR entry). For placenta abruption, work as for Bleeding.

Pre-eclampsia and hypertension

This indicates a failure of Kidney energy, often linked with Liver energy rising (headaches, dizziness and heat, abdominal tightness) (Girdle Vessel) and Spleen energy failing to descend.

This then affects the Heart. It is useful to work even in extreme cases, provided the mother is under observation in hospital.

Work the Kidney, Conception Vessel and Governing Vessel, palming downwards from GV-20 to the Uterus. Palm up from KI-1. Work the Spleen legs up. Work the Girdle Vessel, Heart–Uterus, Kidney–Uterus and Penetrating Vessel.

Work to release the neck and shoulders.

Work GB-20 with the focus on sending energy down to lower blood pressure.

Work LV-3, if at term, to bring wood energy down.

Prolapse of internal organs

Work the Spleen and Governing Vessel to draw up energy.

Work BL-32 for prolapse of the anus and uterus; it stimulates Ki to go up. GV-20 draws energy up.

Ribflare

Use gentle stretches for the arms and chest. Use side stretches, to open the middle burner.

Bladder 17 opens the chest and BL-18 benefits the middle burner.

Symphysis pubis, diastasis, pain

This is due to the Conception Vessel and Girdle Vessel failing to support the pelvis. Work these meridians.

Hold CV/GV to bring energy to the perineum.

CV-2 benefits symphysis pubis.

Stroke the Girdle Vessel, to draw energy to the front, to the symphysis pubis.

Sacral drawing together.

Urine – retention of, infections

This can be related to the Spleen, Kidney or Bladder – work these meridians, and Kidney–Uterus.

GV-20 and ST-36 tonifiy and raise Ki, BL-28 supports the function of the Bladder, BL-32 resolves dampness as well as clearing heat.

CV-3–5 regulate Bladder.

SP-6 helps with Bladder.

BL-39 and BL-40 help with urination.

Varicose veins

These are caused by the Spleen not holding Blood in the vessels.

Work the Spleen but put no direct pressure over the varicose veins. You can include the lymphatic work under 'leg oedema' to support venous return and any accompanying oedema (note any precautions in the oedema section).

Pre-labour

With all pre-labour work, whether to change the baby's position or to induce labour, it is important to support the mother's connection with her baby. This includes the Heart–Uterus, Kidney–Uterus, Girdle Vessel and abdominal work. Often, energy may be blocked in the mother's sacrum and working BL-32–34, the buttock point and sacral releases will help free this energy. Sometimes neck work will free the spine and sacrum.

Breech

Begin around 32–34 weeks. The main work is on BL-67 – use warming techniques such as rubbing. Do this up to five times a day, for as long as is comfortable (a few minutes at a time). You can also work the whole Bladder meridian in the back and legs.

It is effective to show this to partners.

Work all toes and the feet.

Combine with all fours, knee to chest and bridging positions.

Fetal positioning, optimal

For posterior, oblique or transverse lie use the same type of work as for breech. Show partners.

Induction

Use the main points that are contraindicated in pregnancy, i.e. LI-4, GB-21, SP-6, LV-3, BL-60. Work as strongly and as long as you can. Use any combination. Show parents how to work the ones that bring the most reaction and advise them to work them as long and as often as they feel is beneficial.

Do strong sacral work using BL-31–34.

If you have more time, you can include calming work for relaxation – breathing, Heart–Uterus, Kidney–Uterus, Bladder and Kidney in the back.

Labour

With all labour work, continue to include work that supports the mother's connection with her baby. This work includes Heart–Uterus, Kidney–Uterus, Girdle Vessel and abdominal work.

Any stage of labour

Baby – distress   Ensure the flow of Ki, Blood and Essence. Work particularly the Heart–Uterus, Kidney–Uterus, Girdle Vessel, HP-8, CV-4.

Baby – position   If the baby is in an unsuitable position, then freeing energy and balancing Kyo and Jitsu in the sacrum, especially BL-31–34, and neck, especially GB-20, BL-10, GV-15/16 and the five-point head hold, will help the baby to move. The Bladder stimulates movement of the baby so work the Bladder legs and sacrum, especially BL-67 and BL-60. The Girdle Vessel helps to free the energy of the pelvis which may help the baby to move.

If the baby is stuck over one side, it often shows in one side of the sacrum or neck being more Jitsu.

If the baby's head is high, work to bring energy down, especially GB-21 and LV-3, and work down the Governing Vessel and Bladder in the neck and legs.

Mother

Breathing support   Use abdominal holds, especially the Girdle Vessel. Do Lung work, especially L-7. Palming down the Bladder.

Diarrhoea   LI-4.

Exhaustion/blanking out   This is usually due to depletion of Kidney and Yang energy. Work the Bladder/Kidney/Governing Vessel in the back down to the Uterus, stroking or holding. Work the Kidney–Uterus. ST-36, GV-20 and KI-1 all help with exhaustion.

Fear/anxiety   This is often related to fire or water energy. Work the Kidney/Bladder/Governing Vessel back. Work the Bladder down the legs to the feet. Feet holding. Hand holding. Heart and Heart Protector. Include KI-1, HP-8 and BL-60 for calming emotions.

Relaxation – promoting Holding or stroking the Bladder/Kidney/Governing Vessel. GV-20, KI-1 and HP-8 are all calming.

Retention of urine See earlier entry in the Pregnancy section.

Sickness and vomiting LI-4, HP-6.

Tension in the neck/pain relief for the neck Bladder/Gall Bladder neck. Work BL-10, GB-20 and GV-20, GV-15/14, the five-point hold.

Tension or lack of energy in the back/pain relief for the back Use sacrum holds and points, the buttock point, Bladder, Kidney, Girdle Vessel and Governing Vessel meridians. BL-60.

Tension in the shoulders/pain relief Use the three-point hold, stroking techniques, leaning and GB-21.

Trembly legs Use GB-30 and GB-31, BL-60, Bladder and Gall Bladder meridians. The leg stroking technique.

First stage

Throughout, you need to support the flow of water, i.e. Kidney, Bladder and Governing Vessel/ Conception Vessel, using sacral, coccyx and neck holds. Focus on working down the legs. With all situations, try as much as possible to see where there is too much energy and where there is not enough and balance it.

Cervix Swelling – CV-3.

Tight, failing to dilate – GB-34.

Contractions Ineffective, irregular, stopping – GB-21, LV-3, SP-6, BL-60, BL-67, LI-4, CV-4.

Girdle vessel, Kidney–Uterus. Release from sacrum.

Transition If it is because the wood energy is stuck (the mother will be expressing anger, irritability, tight shoulders) use GB-21, GB-20, relax the jaw through opening, release the neck and shoulders, bring energy to the abdomen through holds and to the perineum with the CV/GV hold.

If it is because the water energy is stuck the mother will be fearful, or feel tired or spaced out, labour may stop, she may go quiet, there feels no energy – work to bring energy to the back

through the Governing Vessel, Bladder, Kidney and use BL-67, BL-60, BL-10, KI-1, GV-20.

Urge to bear down when cervix is incompletely dilated Draw up the GV hold with an upwards focus on GV-20. You can also work up the Governing Vessel or Conception Vessel.

Second stage

Ensure that wood energy is flowing – often you will need to work to release tightness in the shoulders, jaw and neck and to bring energy/focus to the perineum GV/CV hold.

Increase the downward movement of Yang by working down the Governing Vessel and working from back to front of the Girdle Vessel. Downwards focus on GV-20.

Stimulate second-stage contractions Use GB-21 especially, also LV-3, but you can then try other induction points.

Aid descent of baby GB-21, LV-3.

Focus mother's attention on the perineum GV/CV hold.

Third stage

Retained placenta First try GB-21, then LV-3, LI-4. Then CV-3, CV-4, CV-6 and BL-60.

Haemorrhage/bleeding Work up the Spleen and Governing Vessel to draw Blood energy upwards.

BL-32 stimulates Ki to move upwards.

CV-3–5, SP-1, LV-1, BL-34 and SP-6 all help with uterine bleeding.

Shock This affects fire energy.

Work the Heart–Uterus, Heart Protector arm. Hand holds. Foot holds to bring energy down.

HT-7, HP-8.

Postnatal – mother

Remember, in the early postnatal period energy is depleted. Shiatsu involves a lot of holding work. For conditions that may also arise in pregnancy, see the relevant condition in the pregnancy section.

Abdominal pain, afterpains

This is often caused by imbalances in Blood energy. You need to work to balance the Heart–Uterus,

Penetrating Vessel, Stomach and Spleen, Conception Vessel.

If there is more general pain and tiredness, then include gentle palming and holding of the abdomen with the Girdle Vessel.

If the pain is more to do with excessive uterine contractions or the uterus not contracting, then include GB-21.

SP-6 helps with abdominal pain.

Bonding

To promote bonding, work the Heart Protector, Heart–Uterus and encourage the mother to do some baby shiatsu.

Constipation

This is usually due to a lack of fluids, which includes Blood. Work with the Conception Vessel, Stomach, Liver (to move Blood).

LV-8 nourishes Liver Blood.

LU-7 and KI-6 regulate the Conception Vessel which nourishes Yin and body fluids.

ST-36 and SP-6 tonify Ki and Blood.

BL-25 stimulates the intestines.

Depression

The Heart meridian is one of the most important to consider, but other organs/meridians than the Heart may be involved. Consider also the Liver, Kidney and Penetrating Vessels (as it is the Sea of Blood).

GV-20 lifts mood.

CV-4 nourishes Blood and strengthens Uterus.

ST-36 and SP-6 nourish the Blood.

HP-6 calms the mind.

KI-1 calms the mind.

Exhaustion

This is often related to depletion of the Kidney energy, Essence and Yin. Work the Kidney–Uterus, Governing, Conception and Penetrating Vessels, balancing Bladder points in the back.

Fever

Do not over-work but it may be useful to support Yin – work the Conception Vessel, especially with holding techniques.

Lactation and breasts

Relax and release the neck and shoulders. Work on and around the breasts.

If the problem is to do with insufficient milk (i.e. Blood) then work with the Penetrating Vessel and Stomach.

If the problem is to do with milk being blocked in the ducts, or the flow of milk, then work the Gall Bladder and Liver and lymph pump to help with the movement of Ki.

ST-36 and SP-6 benefit Ki and Blood.

ST-18 and ST-12 influence energy flows in the breast.

BL-20 and BL-23 tonify Ki and Blood.

CV-17 tonifies Ki in the chest.

GB-34 and LV-3 move Ki.

GB-21 moves Liver Ki.

TH-3 moves Ki and removes obstructions from the upper burner.

Lochia

Focus on the Blood energy – the Penetrating Vessel, Conception Vessel, Stomach, Spleen, Heart–Uterus.

If it feels like it is stuck, i.e. leaking out with clots, then focus on helping energy to flow out and down. Work down the legs to the feet. ST-36 helps to draw energy down.

If it feels like a lot of pale blood loss, then you want to strengthen Blood energy – the Penetrating Vessel point combination is good for this, GV-20 to raise energy up, SP-1 to stop uterine bleeding.

If there is infection i.e. bright red, dark red, with a foul smell, work gently and don't focus on moving energy away. Gentle holding of the abdomen and Uterus is better.

CV-12, CV-6, SP-6 all benefit Blood.

CV-4 is an important point to nourish Blood, strengthen Uterus and tonify the Conception Vessel and Penetrating Vessel.

BL-17 benefits Blood.

Perineum

Holding CV-1 and GV-2 helps with energy flows through the perineum and promotes healing.

Postnatal – baby

Generally, gently stroking and holding all the meridians is of benefit. It does not take long to work the whole baby's body.

Chest infections/mucous

Spleen and Lung. L-1 and L-2.

Colic

Trauma to the nervous system expresses itself as colic – this is not primarily a digestive system problem. Work on the Heart Protector as well as the Stomach and Intestines is important in these situations.

Use clockwise abdominal massage, nourishing Kyo areas and easing out Jitsu areas (there are often many areas of hardness). Work the feet to bring energy down.

CV-12 regulates Stomach.
ST-36 regulates Stomach.
HP-6 calms energy.

Constipation

Babies don't have bowel movements every day, but if they have hard stools or seem to be straining, then they may be constipated. Gentle shiatsu can be done on the abdomen and around the anus.

BL-25 and ST-25 benefit Large Intestine.

Eczema

Work the Stomach and Spleen on the legs and the Lung arms.

Reluctant feeders

This is often due to Stomach energy not reaching forward. Work the Stomach face, chest and legs.

If the baby is unsettled, then work the Stomach and Heart Protector arms to settle fire energy.

ST-36 helps to regulate Stomach and settle energy.

HP-8 is a calming point.

Sleeplessness

This is often due to restlessness in the baby's fire energy.

Work the Heart Protector in the arms and the Stomach and Spleen legs to ground and settle.

Work the Governing Vessel and Bladder back and legs to calm the active Yang.

If it seems more like a digestive or colic pattern, then focus more on the Spleen Stomach and work on the abdomen and feet.

HP-8 and KI-1 are calming.
ST-36 is grounding.
CV-12 regulates Stomach.
ST-36 helps with digestion.

Traumatized babies

Use simple head holding and work with the Governing Vessel head and back – especially for forceps/ventouse/Caesarean-delivered babies. If it feels too much, then do it with the same intention and connections but a short way off the body.

Vomit

Use the points as for colic, plus ST-34 and BL-21 regulate Stomach.

Please refer to Appendix 3 for further information on matters relating to safety and diagnosis issues.

REFERENCES

Chamberlain D 1988 Babies remember birth and other extraordinary scientific discoveries about the mind and personality of your newborn. Jeremey Tarcher, USA

Janov A 1983 Imprints: the lifelong effects of the birth experience. Coward-McCann, New York

Noble E 1993 Primal connections: how our experiences from conception to birth influence our emotions, behaviour and health. Simon Schuster, New York

Verny T R 1992 Obstetrical procedures: a critical examination of their effect on pregnant women and their unborn and newborn children. Pre and Perinatal Psychology Journal 7:101–112

Shiatsu for self-healing

This section explores the different ways in which shiatsu can be used to support the well-being of midwives and to enable their work with women to be most effective. It considers the use of shiatsu exercise, as well as touch techniques, which can be done on oneself and the benefits of receiving shiatsu from a practitioner.

8

Using shiatsu to heal yourself

Introduction

'Physician heal thyself'

This age-old adage is fundamental for anyone working with shiatsu. For shiatsu to be at its most effective and for midwives to feel comfortable while doing shiatsu, they need to have worked with balancing their own energy, as much as they can. The benefits of this will show themselves not only in better shiatsu, but also in feeling better in oneself. Shiatsu is a great tool for helping to prevent burnout and stress, which is especially relevant in today's pressurized working conditions.

The best ways of doing this are:

- Working with exercises to ensure the flow of energy through your meridians. Some exercises have already been described in Chapter 5. In this chapter I present some additional exercises, which are primarily aimed at the midwife but can also be adapted for pregnant women. If you feel that a woman would particularly benefit from one or more of these exercises and that you are competent to teach them, some guidelines are given on how to adapt them.
- Doing 'self-shiatsu' on some of the meridians and points.
- Receiving regular shiatsu sessions. Receiving shiatsu is a good way of learning about shiatsu, as well as balancing one's own energy.

Self-healing exercises

Ki exercises – the Makkho

One of the 'fathers' of modern shiatsu – Shitzuko Masunaga – developed a series of exercises which he called the Zen imagery exercises. He expounds on these exercises in an excellent book called Zen Imagery Exercises (Masunaga 1987). While all the exercises are useful, a basic series of six exercises known as the Makkho exercises is widely taught on most shiatsu courses. Each shiatsu school seems to teach a slightly different variation. I will describe the version with which I feel most comfortable working.

Each exercise balances a pair of the 12 main meridians. Practised daily, they balance Ki in the body. They are similar to yoga postures. In fact, studying Masunaga's book you will see that many more of the exercises resemble yoga. One American teacher, Michael Reed Gach, developed a whole system called Acu Yoga based on the links between the meridians and yoga (Reed Gach 1981). There are many similarities between yoga and shiatsu. This is not surprising since both developed in the East and there was a great exchange of ideas between China, Japan and India.

Many Westerners find some of these exercises quite challenging at first – but if you work with them they should all feel easier as you free up energy flows in your body. Energy includes your physical structure of muscles and ligaments which initially may be tight. You have to remember that these exercises were developed by Masunaga in Japan in the 1970s and the Japanese tend to be more flexible than Westerners. Even though, in post-war Japan, there has been a shift away from the traditional practices of health and healing, the Japanese still often sit in the seiza position. This is where you sit with your legs folded under your hips and is similar to the starting position for the Stomach/Spleen exercise (see later in this chapter). This means that Japanese people tend to have more flexible hips and find the exercises easier. It is often difficult for Westerners to feel comfortable in seiza unless they have done a lot of yoga-style exercise.

It is important to only move in the exercise to the point where you feel a stretch – which may

well not be the full stretch position. It can vary considerably from person to person, depending on the individual flexibility. The exercises are a good self-diagnostic tool. If you work with each exercise and feel which is the easiest and which is the hardest, you are finding which is your most Kyo (lacking in energy) and which is your most Jitsu (too much energy) meridian. Practising these exercises, you will also begin to build up a clearer picture of where the meridians run and the effects of different meridians on your body.

Box 8.1

- Do you think the easiest exercise represents the most Kyo or Jitsu meridian?
- Do you think that there will be differences depending on the time of day you do the exercises? If so, what and why?

Beginning the exercises, we must first of all begin by being aware of our breathing. Breath is an important form of Ki, and breathing more deeply helps the Ki to flow better and makes the exercises more effective.

Begin by standing and doing the hara breathing exercise (see p. 74), in the standing position. When you are breathing deeply, you are ready to begin the exercises.

With all these exercises, breathe out as you move, and move slowly only as far as you feel comfortable. While holding a position, focus on the out-breath and on feeling what is going on in your body. Feel that you are allowing energy to flow through you. Be aware of any sensations, both physical and emotional. For most of these exercises you need to stay for at least three out-breaths in the final position, but then, if you feel you are tensing and that energy is not flowing, you need to come out of the position slowly. There should be no strong discomfort in any position, although sometimes you may be aware of stretching or a mild ache as you work parts of your body that you are not used to using. If, however, at any point you feel sharp pain, then immediately come out of the position slowly. It is important not to strain. If, on the other hand, you are comfortable and relaxed, continue to stay in the position for a while longer. By staying as long as you feel is right in each position, you are balancing the Kyo and the Jitsu. The Kyo needs you to stay longer to enable energy to flow to it and the Jitsu needs more movement to enable it to shift.

You may want to integrate these exercises with the element meditations from Chapters 6 and 7.

The most effective way of working with these exercises is to go through the whole sequence twice and to do them daily. The first time we are often only releasing physical stiffness and not working at a deep level. The second time round, the effect is more profound. If, however, you have less time, then you can do the whole sequence once and then simply repeat the most Kyo exercise followed by the most Jitsu exercise. If you have even less time, on some occasions, once you know your patterns and which tend to be your most Kyo and most Jitsu exercises, then you can focus on those two. It is better to try to go through the whole sequence at least once if you are able. It is best if you can find a regular time of day to do them. If you do them at different times, you will probably find that different exercises are Kyo and Jitsu. This reflects the different peaks of flow of energy in the meridians.

I give suggestions on how to adapt the exercises in pregnancy. They are suitable postnatally but not in the early postnatal period when other exercises would be more suitable. It is outside the scope of this book to discuss early postnatal exercises in detail.

The order of the exercises is important as it follows the daily flow of energy through the meridians.

Makkho 1 – Lung and Large Intestine

As you would expect, this is especially good for opening the chest and clearing the lungs, as well as stretching the back of the legs.

Stand upright with your feet about hip width apart and your feet slightly turned in. Take your hands behind your back and link your two thumbs together and touch your two index fingers together. If this feels uncomfortable, you can link all fingers together. The Lung flows through the thumb (L-11) and the Large Intestine through the index finger (LI-1). As you breathe out, open your chest by squeezing your shoulder blades

together and extending your arms (Fig. 8.1A). Breathe deeply in this position for a few breaths. On another out-breath, lean forwards, keeping your arms linked and extended and your knees relaxed but not bent or locked. Lean as far as you can without straining (Fig. 8.1B). Relax your head. Allow your arms to move as far forward as is comfortable. Stay for a minimum of three

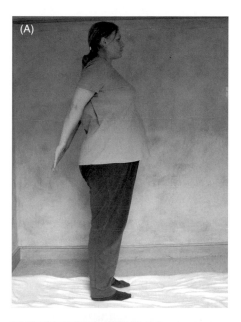

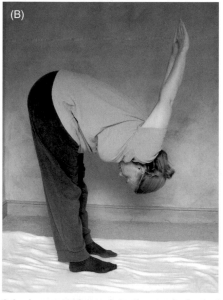

Figure 8.1   Lung and Large Intestine work. A: start position and B: bending.

out-breaths, but come up, on an out-breath, when you feel you have held it long enough. After a few deep out-breaths, repeat twice more.

In pregnancy   Some women may be comfortable all the way through their pregnancy doing this exercise, although as their abdomen gets bigger, they may not be able to go down so far. Other women may find that they feel dizzy as they go down and therefore they should just concentrate on the first part of the exercise.

Makkho 2 – Stomach and Spleen

This one is the most challenging of the exercises, as many people find even the starting position difficult. This is like the seiza position.

Begin by kneeling, sitting between your heels, ideally with your bottom on the floor and knees as close together as is comfortable. Seiza is sitting with your heels into your buttocks. If this is not comfortable then you can sit on your heels but then do not attempt the rest of the exercise. Simply kneeling in this position is already working the meridians. People with knee injuries may well find this exercise is not possible to do at all, if it feels like it is straining the knees. If this is the case, then do not do it.

It is important in this exercise that you use your arms and not your back to lower yourself down and to ease yourself up.

Place your hands on your feet so that you can hold on to them as you gradually use your forearms to ease backwards towards the ground as far as you can. Be careful not to feel strain in your lower back. If you can comfortably rest your upper back on the ground without strain on your lower back, then you can stretch out your arms behind your head (Fig. 8.2). Stay as long as you can in whatever position is comfortable, breathing out deeply and relaxing into any areas where you feel a stretch.

When you are ready to come up, have your hands holding your feet and use your forearms to ease you back to kneeling.

If you find this version difficult, you can adapt this by leaning back against a chair or cushions so that your back is more supported and you don't go so far back (Fig. 8.3).

In pregnancy   The full exercise is obviously not suitable for pregnant women as it places too

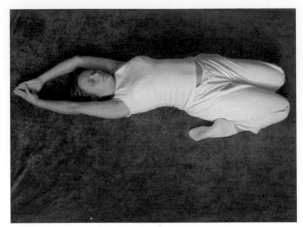

Figure 8.2   Stomach and Spleen.

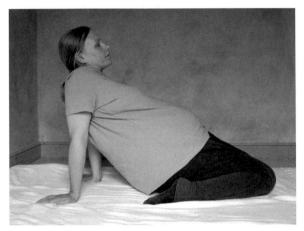

Figure 8.3   Stomach and Spleen adaptation.

much strain on the lower back and abdomen. You can do the kneeling without leaning back. You can lean a short way back as in Fig. 8.3. Another version is to stand on both feet. Bend one leg behind you and hold the back of your foot with the hand on the same side. Ease the heel towards the buttock but don't force it. Try to keep your knees as close together as you can. Now lift your other hand towards the shoulder on the same side with the palm facing forward and then stretch it above your head. Hold it for a little while, breathing deeply. Then, ease the leg down and, after a short pause, repeat on the other side.

This is especially good for opening the front of the body and for rib flare and carpal tunnel syndrome.

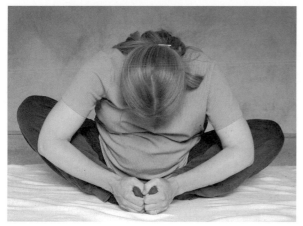

Figure 8.4   Heart and Small Intestine.

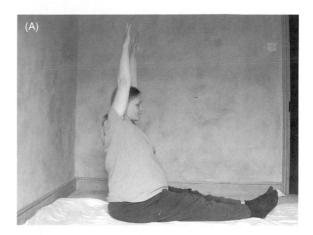

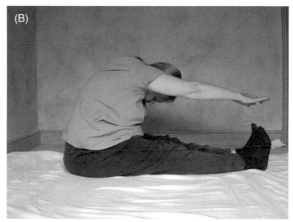

Figure 8.5   Bladder and Kidney.

Makkho 3 – Heart and Small Intestine

Sit with the soles of your feet together and allow your hips to relax. Hold onto your feet with your hands and bend your arms at the elbow and away from your body. As you breathe out, ease forward, bringing your forearms towards the ground in front of your legs (Fig. 8.4). Allow your neck to relax. Breathe out for at least three out-breaths in this position. When you are ready, slowly ease back to sitting by uncurling your back from the bottom up.

In pregnancy   Little adaptation needs to be made for this, except if the mother has symphysis pubis diastasis, in which case the exercise would not be suitable. As the pregnancy progresses, the mother will find she will not be able to go so far forward, but it can often remain a comfortable position until the end.

Makkho 4 – Bladder and Kidney

This exercise follows what the body naturally wants to do after the Heart/Small Intestine – that is to stretch out your legs. Remaining sitting, extend your legs so that they are straight and together, and slightly ease your toes towards your body to stretch the backs of your legs.

Next, lift your hands to the side of each shoulder so that you open up your upper back. Then, as you breathe out, extend your arms above your head, parallel to each other and in line with the side of your body (Fig. 8.5A). Feel the stretch in your back, in the spine and down each side of the spine. As you breathe out, relax, and as you breathe in, feel the spine extending, almost as though you have a piece of string attached to the top of your head pulling you upwards. Don't slouch. You want to keep this feeling of extension in the back as you breathe out again and ease forward, keeping your spine and arms extended, feeling as though you are hinging from the hips (Fig. 8.5B). Ease down as far as you are comfortable. If you can touch your toes, hold onto your little toes and, if you can, place your other fingers just below the ball of the foot. Breathe out for at least three out-breaths in this position. When you want to come up, ease up on your out-breath, again hinging from your hips, and keeping your spine and arms extended. After one time, you can either continue when you are ready or bring your arms back down for a short rest. Repeat three times.

In pregnancy This exercise may be helpful in pregnancy – of course, as the baby gets bigger the mother will not be able to lean so far forward, but she can still feel the movement of energy along the back and the backs of the legs. It is often an excellent exercise for women with symphysis pubis diastasis as it strengthens the energy of the midline of the body without placing pressure on the symphysis pubis.

Makkho 5 – Heart Protector and Triple Heater

If you are able to sit in the half lotus position with one foot onto your inner thigh and then bringing the other foot across and onto the thigh of the already bent leg, then begin in this way. If you are not able to do this, then sit cross legged. Next, cross your arms, bringing them close in to your body and placing the back of your hands on your opposite thighs (Fig. 8.6). As you breathe out, ease as far forward as you can, keeping your arms into your body, without allowing your bottom to lift off the ground. Relax your neck and, if your head can rest on the ground, allow it to do so.

Repeat three times. You can then repeat a further three times if you wish, crossing the legs and the arms in the opposite way.

In pregnancy This is often comfortable. As the mother gets bigger, she may want to place her crossed arms, with palms up, over a cushion in front of her, so she doesn't have to lean so far forward. This is not suitable for women with SPD.

Makkho 6 – Gall Bladder and Liver

Sit and bend one leg so that the foot comes onto the thigh of the other leg. Have the other leg extended. Extend your arms to the side and then twist your hips so that your arms are parallel to the ground and in line with your hips and the extended leg. You are facing your bent knee. As you breathe out, ease towards the side with the extended leg, keeping your hips in line with your arms. If you can reach and hold the ankle or toes of the foot of the extended leg, then do so. With the other arm, ease your shoulders back and look up to the hand (Fig. 8.7).

In pregnancy This exercise is often easier in pregnancy, because of the effects of relaxin and progesterone, softening the ligaments. It is very

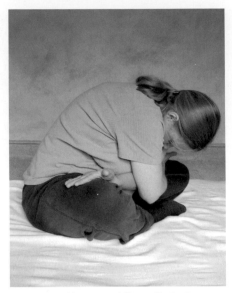
Figure 8.6 Triple Heater and Heart Protector.

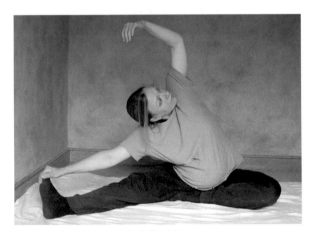
Figure 8.7 Liver and Gall Bladder.

beneficial for stretching the side of the body and the neck and the shoulders, and freeing up the wood energy which tends to get stuck. It is not suitable for women with SPD.

Case study 8.1 Jill, community midwife, the Borders, Scotland

Working with makkho was a very positive experience in that I was beginning to gain confidence with the flow of these exercises, I was feeling more familiar with the regime, the posture/positioning, and felt growing relaxation, escapism, well-being, a sense of stillness but yet one of total re-energizing/something just for me.

I was building on the growing confidence and feeling of well-being that is derived from the makkho exercises, along with re-energizing myself and restoring balance to my own energy flow in order that my physical and emotional equilibrium would be optimal for practising shiatsu.

It was clear, working through the exercises that, as familiarization and confidence grows, it will be a most valuable 'working/timeout' tool for use both in the working and the domestic setting.

Case study 8.2   Julie, senior midwifery lecturer at the University of the West of England, Bristol

Trying to do the makkho exercises to stretch the meridians was quite salutary for me when I discovered that I found most of them very hard and quite uncomfortable to do. For someone who prides herself on keeping fit, it was a bit of a shock to find I was really stiff and inflexible! Needless to say, despite good intentions, I haven't kept them up, although I do feel the benefit of them when I do them. This course has made me realize the importance of listening to, and tuning into, one's own body as well as those of one's clients. Without an awareness of both, it is impossible to provide effective shiatsu treatment. Perhaps this awareness should also be a fundamental aspect of midwifery practice.

Essence exercises – the Well Mother approach

This is a sequence of exercises I have developed over my years of antenatal and postnatal teaching. They draw on my blending together of yoga and shiatsu, and my understanding of the importance of the extraordinary vessels and the energy of the Essence in pregnancy. Since they are working on Essence, they are a useful back-up to the Makkho exercises. In fact, Masunaga developed a series of exercises for the Conception Vessel and Governing Vessel, but his exercises are not so suited to pregnancy. The exercises I have developed are all potentially suitable for pregnant women to do and can be worked towards in the later postnatal period. They are also beneficial for women who are not pregnant. They can be especially useful for menopausal women, for whom the Essence is declining and there are shifts in energy flow to and from the uterus.

I present these here, partly for your own self-healing, but also because you may well recognize versions of many of these exercises. By doing

them, you can become more aware of the energy of the Governing, Conception and Penetrating Vessels and understand how, with a shift of focus, many exercises you may already show women can also benefit the Governing, Conception and Penetrating Vessels. It is up to you to decide how competent you are to teach these exercises.

It is helpful to do these everyday, like the Makkho, if you have time. You may find that you prefer to do these in the evening and the Makkho in the morning or vice versa. You may find that some days you prefer to do these and other days the Makkho.

Before beginning these, it is important to work with hara breathing (p. 74). They don't necessarily have to be done in a particular order, as they are all working with the extraordinary vessels (Governing Vessel, Conception Vessel and Penetrating Vessel). However, it is usually best to begin either with the standing exercise or the all fours and to finish with one of the lying ones. Of course, later in pregnancy, the lying-down ones may not be possible to do, so then the mother just needs to rest on her side, or on all fours.

With all of these, you want to focus on the flow of energy along the Conception/Penetrating Vessel meridian at the front of the body and the Governing Vessel at the back.

All fours movements

Crawling   We can begin with the crawling posture i.e. on hands and knees. Remember the crawling from the basic shiatsu exercises or turn now to read (on p. 76). Crawl around for a while, keeping the lower back flat. From crawling come to resting in all fours. Then begin to rock gently forwards and backwards. If you are comfortable as you go forwards, allow your hips to drop and your feet to come off the ground. As you go back, you may sit back on your heels and allow your head to rest on the floor. The breath doesn't need to be focused on any particular part of this movement, but do make sure you are breathing slowly. As you rock, be aware of the lines of energy down the front and back of your body.

After a few minutes, come to rest in the all fours position.

The cat   This is similar to the cat in yoga, although the breathing and part of the movement

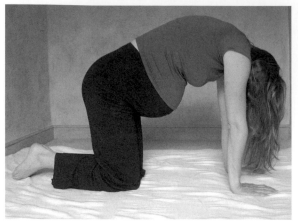

Figure 8.8   In the extended position of the cat.

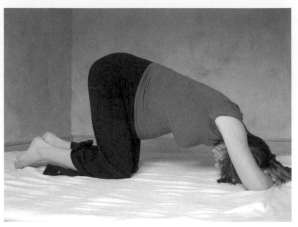

Figure 8.9   Knee to chest.

may be slightly different, depending on the tradition of yoga. In the all fours position, make sure that your back is flat, so you may need to slightly bend your elbows, to bring your upper back in line with your lower back. As you breathe out, slowly lower your head towards the ground, without bending your arms any more. As you continue to breathe out, push down into your hands, extend your arms and slowly begin to lift and round your spine, like a cat arching its back (Fig. 8.8). At the end of the out-breath, feel the rounding of the lower back and the drawing in of your abdominals. As you breathe in, flatten and extend the spine, beginning with the base of the spine and working to the neck, to finish in the starting flat-back position. Your neck needs to be in line with your spine. Repeat this series of movements for several minutes, lifting and rounding the spine on the in-breath, and flattening and extending the spine on the out-breath. As you repeat these movements, focus on the pathways of the CV/PV and GV.

When you have finished, you can rest in one of the two following positions:

1. Knee to chest   Place your forearms onto the ground and bring them towards you so that each hand is on the elbow of the opposite arm. Lower your chest towards the ground. Rest your head where it is most comfortable but lower than your bottom. Make sure that your spine is flat. Breathe into your hara and rest in this position for a few minutes (Fig. 8.9).

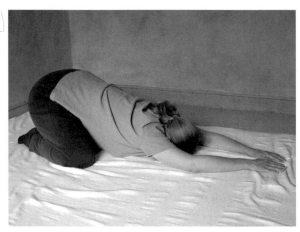

Figure 8.10   Swan.

2. Swan   Sit back down on your heels. If you are pregnant you will need to open out your knees a little. Slide your arms along the ground so that they are extended in front of you. Rest your head on the ground where it is comfortable (Fig. 8.10). Try to have your whole spine as flat as you can. Breathe out into your hara and rest in this position for a few minutes.

Squat

You can ease towards the squatting position by pushing backwards into a kneeling position and rocking back onto your toes. Alternatively, you can begin by assuming a semi-squatting position. Place your hands on the floor in front of you. Before going into the full squat, gently rock from

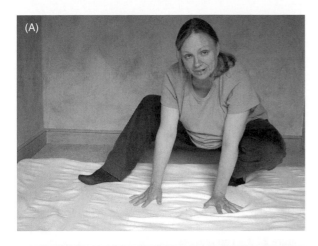

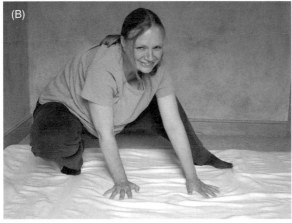

Figure 8.11 A and B: The rocking squat.

side to side for a few minutes. You do this by pivoting your hips so you bring one knee towards the ground in front of you, with the heel off the ground. The foot of the other leg is flat on the ground, shin and thigh at approximately 45°. Repeat to the other side with a continuous rocking movement (Fig. 8.11A and B).

When you feel your legs are prepared, you can ease into the full squat. Have your feet as close together or as far apart as feels comfortable. Ideally, you want to have your feet flat on the ground and your weight in the centre of the foot.

If you are not able to do this then you can either:

- hold onto a door handle
- put some blocks or books under your heels
- try squatting with a partner.

Partner squatting

Stand facing a partner with your arms extended. Hold hands. As you both breathe out, together ease down to a squat. You need to continue to have your arms extended. Refer back to p. 104.

While you are squatting, focus on the lower part of the CV/PV/GV, i.e. the perineum.

In pregnancy There are various schools of thought on the importance and safety of the squat in pregnancy. I believe that if women start early on, probably towards the beginning of the second trimester, they will probably find it fairly comfortable with a little practice. Some women find it becomes their preferred resting position. It is in the last trimester that more care needs to be taken. If the mother has varicose veins then she should not squat for more than a minute because otherwise she may block the flow of blood. If she has haemorrhoids, it will probably be uncomfortable to squat at all. If the baby is in breech, then she should not squat until the baby has turned, because squatting will make the bottom engage more, although, when the baby has turned, squatting will help the baby stay cephalic. If the baby is transverse or oblique, then squatting will probably not feel comfortable. If the baby is posterior, then more time should be spent on all fours than in the squat, but the squat should not necessarily be avoided entirely. Women with symphysis pubis diastasis should not squat at all because it strains the joint. Women with some types of knee injuries may find squatting places too much strain on the knee – in which case they should not squat. The key factor is that, while it may feel challenging, it should not feel painful.

Squat to standing

From your squat, as you breathe out, have your arms extended so that they are parallel to the ground and push down in your feet so that you use the strength in your legs to bring you to standing, and not your back (Fig. 8.12).

Once in the standing position, relax your arms by your sides, breathe out and rest for a few out-breaths. As you breathe out, feel the weight of your feet on the ground. Be aware of the movement of your spine on the in-breath. Feel as though there

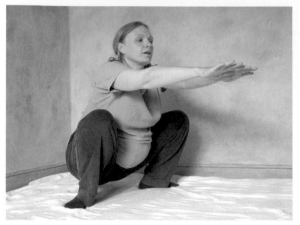

Figure 8.12 Squatting to standing, using legs not back.

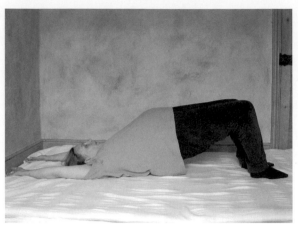

Figure 8.13 The bridge.

is a piece of string attaching the top of your head (GV-20) to the ceiling. As you breathe out, relax, and as you breathe in, feel this thread extending. After a while, slowly lift the heels of your feet away from the ground so that you feel some movement of energy in your legs, while still keeping your toes and the ball of your foot on the floor. Make sure that your lower back is flat and not arching, so your pelvis will be tilted slightly back. Bring your hands to your shoulders, keeping your upper arm close into your body (like in the beginning of the Bladder/Kidney Makkho) and then extend your hands above your head in line with your spine. Make sure that your back is flat, especially the upper back. If your upper back is very rounded, you may need to relax your arms and ease your shoulders back to flatten the upper back. Feel the thread extending through your spine, as you breathe. As you breathe out, relax your neck and shoulders without moving their position. When you feel that you have held this for long enough, after several minutes, slowly ease back down to the starting position, bringing your arms to rest along the sides of your body and your feet back to a flat foot position. Stay resting for a minute or so in this position and be aware of any changes in your body.

After this, slowly bend your knees and begin to curl forwards, bringing your head towards the ground. Just curl as far forwards as is comfortable. Rest curled over for a minute or so, feeling floppy and heavy like a rag doll. On an out-breath,

slowly begin to uncurl from the base of the spine, working up to the top of the spine. You may take several out-breaths to do this. Feel as though you are gently stacking one vertebrae on top of the other. Feel the changing relationship between the front and back of the body.

Rest in the upright position for a few minutes, breathing deeply into your hara.

Going from standing to squatting to lying

From standing, lift your arms upwards in front of you so that they are parallel to the ground. As you breathe out, slowly ease down into the squat. From the squat, move forward onto all fours. From all fours, ease down onto your side. From your side, ease onto your back. On your back, have your feet just in front of your buttocks so that your knees are bent. Have your arms along the side of your body. As you breathe out, allow your lower back to soften into the ground. Then gently push your feet into the ground. On an out-breath, ease your lower back from the ground, gradually working from the bottom of the spine up, to finish in a position resting with your head, shoulders, upper back and feet on the ground and your spine extended as much as is comfortable (Fig. 8.13).

Stay in the extended position as you breathe in and feel the extra extension in the spine. As you breathe out, slowly lower the spine back to the ground from the top vertebrae to the bottom. Rest as you breathe in and then start again with the lifting movement.

Repeat as many times as you feel comfortable.

When you have finished, rest with your knees into your chest and breathe out. After a while, you may want to rock gently from side to side.

Conception/Penetrating/Governing Vessel meditation

Breathing and visualization are another way of 'exercising' the meridians. What we are going to do is to follow with our attention the pathways of the Governing, Penetrating and Conception Vessels. Some people find this easy, others find it takes a lot of practice. When you have done the movements, find a comfortable position to sit in to do this meditation/visualization.

Close your eyes and place both hands over your hara below your navel. As you breathe out, feel the gentle movement of your hands drawing in. Just follow the instructions as best you can. After a while, bring your attention to the area between your two Kidneys – the Ming Men. Keep your attention on this point and be aware of any sensations you feel. After a minute or so, allow your attention to move from here to your uterus. Be aware of your uterus, feel that your attention is right inside it. After a while, move your attention from the uterus following a pathway of energy down to the centre of the perineum. Then follow with your attention the pathways of the Conception Vessel and Penetrating Vessel up the front of your body. They flow together up to the pubic bone and across the top of the pubic bone in a band of energy 4 thumbwidths wide. As your attention moves up through the lower abdomen, the band narrows to 1 thumbwidth wide until it reaches the ribs where it spreads out again to 4 thumbwidths until you get to the clavicle where the pathway flows up the throat and enters into the mouth. Bring your attention now down the internal pathway of the meridians – flowing inside your mouth, throat and dropping down deep inside your body to the space between the Kidneys. From here, allow your attention to flow to the uterus and out onto the perineum, and from here up through the anus, the coccyx and all the vertebrae up to the top of the head – the Governing Vessel – over the top of the head and to the mouth. Now, follow your attention inside the mouth to go down the throat and down back

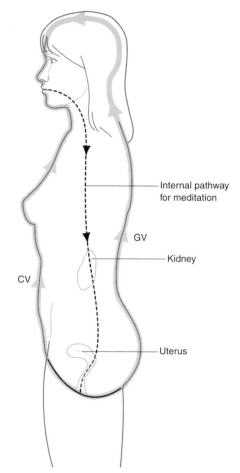

Internal pathway for meditation

GV

Kidney

CV

Uterus

Figure 8.14 Diagram of pathways for meditation.

to the space between the Kidneys. Keep following this circuit of energy for at least several minutes. Finish by being aware of the flow of energy through the uterus (Fig. 8.14).

Partner exercises

These are relaxing and fun to practice with another midwife. They are another way of working with meridians and energy. See pages 75–77.

Self-work on some of the meridians and points

In Japan there has always been the tradition of working on yourself – most shiatsu books give some guidance on how to do this. Essentially, it is simply about applying all the same basic principles and of course it is easy to tell how much pressure to use and how long to stay. It is tempting to focus only on the areas of Jitsu – for example, if we have a stiff neck and shoulders we want to try to ease the stiffness. Do try to remember to look for Kyo areas and work those first – this can be hard to do for yourself.

Much of the shiatsu in this book is suitable for non-pregnant people, including men. You simply need to read through the techniques and functions of the meridians to see what effect the shiatsu is likely to have. The groups of people who are most likely to benefit from similar work to that presented in this book are pubescent girls and menopausal women. Why do you think that is? The reason is because there are dramatic changes happening in the same systems as in pregnancy – changes in the function of the uterus, changes in hormonal and blood flow, changes in flow of Essence, Ki and Blood. Work with the extraordinary vessels is particularly useful, as is the Heart–Uterus and Kidney–Uterus.

How can this be done on yourself? Refer back to the Heart–Uterus visualization on page 123. This includes some palming down or up the meridian, depending on which organ you feel is most Kyo or Jitsu. With someone suffering from hot flushes, common during the menopause, palming down is often very helpful. It is even the kind of shiatsu that can be done if you wake up in the middle of the night. You can do the same type of work, but focus more on the Conception Vessel or Penetrating Vessel.

Working the combined points (see p. 134) of the extraordinary vessels is effective. You can hold the point in the foot with one hand and with your free hand work the corresponding point on the hand. Remember to do both sides. Working on the hands is quite easy to do. HP-6 and HP-8 are often good for emotional distress (see p. 115). Hold one hand in the other hand, so you have a mother hand, and then place your thumb in the relevant point. Working on the feet or legs is even easier because you have two hands to work. Working on the neck and head can be great if you have been sat at a desk all day and can give good relief. The back is a harder area – but it is possible to access some points. Holding your hands over the two Kidneys and letting your back feel supported can be calming and relaxing. This is something people often do instinctively, and reminds us how shiatsu is one of the most natural and instinctive things to do – once we learn how to connect with it. After holding the Kidneys, you can place one hand over the Uterus and connect with the Kidneys and Uterus. Remember to do both sides.

Don't be afraid to experiment a little – your body will let you know what feels right. You can work on yourself as a way of learning more about shiatsu, but do remember that just because you particularly like or dislike something it doesn't necessarily mean that it will be the same for others because everyone's energy is different.

It is advisable not to work a lot with the points that are contraindicated in pregnancy (see p. 122) as these are very powerful points which shift energy more dramatically than other points. Some women find that they help ease period pains; but if you find that you are using them month after month with no change in the symptoms, then it is best to see a shiatsu practitioner and have a more thorough diagnosis.

Receiving regular shiatsu

For even the most experienced shiatsu practitioner, there can be no substitute for going to see another shiatsu practitioner on a reasonably regular basis (i.e. at least every few months, although once a month if possible is best). Another person can see patterns that you cannot, and it is a time for someone else to focus on balancing your energy.

The midwife could swap sessions with another midwife who has studied shiatsu or she may want to go and see a shiatsu practitioner. By experiencing shiatsu in a context other than maternity, the midwife will learn more about her own energy as well as different ways of touching. She may use it as an opportunity to find which shiatsu practitioners in her area she most feels comfortable referring women to, as well as identifying which shiatsu practitioners she can work with to support her own shiatsu work.

There are many different styles of shiatsu and it is best to try out a few shiatsu practitioners who have trained in different schools and styles and see which you like. You may like to see a male practitioner or you may prefer a woman. Shiatsu is more of an 'art' than a science and how you feel with the practitioner is important. It is unlikely that two practitioners will come up with exactly the same diagnosis – there will be similarities but different practitioners may emphasize different aspects.

Questions to ask a shiatsu practitioner

You may want to ask about the style of shiatsu they do – there are many styles, from the very physical, more like chiropractics, to much lighter styles, more like spiritual healing. You may want to find out about the school they trained with and any particular traditions it embraces. You may want to ask how they would describe their style of shiatsu.

You will probably want to ask some questions about how they make their diagnosis. Do they use pulse and tongue as well as hara and touch diagnosis?

What other work do they do to complement the hands-on work of shiatsu? Some practitioners may emphasize diet, others breathing and exercise, others lifestyle suggestions; some may use herbs and acupuncture alongside shiatsu. Think about what you want from the shiatsu. A practitioner can potentially support you in many areas of your life and you need to think about their individual approach and how it suits you.

You may want to use your own experiences of receiving shiatsu as an opportunity to build up lists of practitioners you feel comfortable referring pregnant women to. Not all practitioners have done much work with pregnant women. Some styles of shiatsu you may feel are less suitable to pregnancy, such as the more physical styles or a 'routine' type of approach. An experienced shiatsu practitioner is able to blend many different styles and offer each client the approach that best suits them – working from the more physical to the more energetic.

REFERENCES

Masunaga S 1987 Zen imagery exercises. Japan Publications, Tokyo
Reed Gach M 1981 Acu-Yoga. Japan Publications, Tokyo

FURTHER READING

Lundberg P 1973 The book of shiatsu. Gaia Books, London
Jarmey C, Mojay G 1999 Shiatsu – the complete guide. Thorsons, London
Kusmirek J 2002 Liquid sunshine – vegetable oils for aromatherapy. Floramicus, Somerset
Meeus C 2001 Secrets of shiatsu. Dorling Kindersley, London
Pooley N 1998 Shiatsu in a nutshell. Element Books, Shaftesbury, Dorset

Appendices

APPENDICES CONTENTS

Appendix 1

Sample leaflet

What is shiatsu?

Shiatsu is a form of bodywork based largely on acupuncture theory which uses pressure and massage techniques, often combined with breathing and exercise.

Midwives already use similar massage techniques as part of their routine care and shiatsu gives more 'focus' to these practices.

A full session can take approximately 1 hour, however, short 5–15 minutes treatments can also be extremely beneficial.

Shiatsu is a non-invasive holistic therapy which has no absolute contraindications. It is therapeutic and pleasurable to the client. As shiatsu induces relaxation, it aids the restoration of a better state of health and well-being.

Sample of a shiatsu legend

Reported benefits associated with Shiatsu

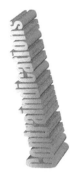

Relaxation

Bonding with baby

Common ailments of pregnancy, e.g. backache, nausea, cramps, oedema, carpal tunnel syndrome

Balancing emotional states

Promoting immunity

Pain relief in labour

Effects in labour, e.g. strengthening contractions

Postnatal ailments, e.g. bleeding, wound healing, depression

Retention of urine

Baby shiatsu

Contraindications

Shiatsu is a non-invasive and relatively safe therapy which works with energy within the body. It does not interact with drugs therefore choices do not need to be made between shiatsu or conventional treatment.

Midwives who have completed the 'Shiatsu skills for Midwives' course are not qualified shiatsu practitioners. However, the training has provided adequate knowledge and skills for midwives to integrate shiatsu into midwifery practice.

Only experienced shiatsu practitioners should work in the following situations:

Infections and inflammation

Severe hypertension and pre-eclampsia

Thrombosis – do not massage leg

Cancer

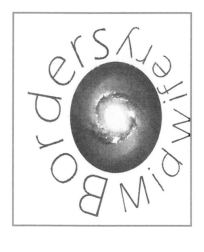

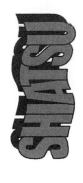

SHIATSU TREATMENT

Midwives who are able to provide shiatsu having completed a **'Shiatsu Skills For Midwives'** course:

Name . . . . Tel . . . .
Name . . . . Tel . . . .
Name . . . . Tel . . . .
Name . . . . Tel . . . .

Any of the above midwives can be contacted for further information if necessary.

I _____
understand the explanation I have been given about shiatsu treatment and agree to be treated by one of the above midwives. I also consent to information being used for audit or research purposes.

Signed..
CRN..

Signed..
Midwife
Date

Initially, if appropriate, shiatsu will be offered to women in the Pregnancy Assessment Unit, Ward 17 or Labour Ward.

References:-
Dunn P A, Roger D, Halford K (1989) Transcutaneous electrical stimulation at acupuncture points in the induction of uterine contractions. *Obstetrics & Gynaecology;* **73**: 286–290

Kubista E et al (1975) Initiating contractions of the gravid uterus through electro-acupuncture. *American Journal of Chinese Medicine;* **3**: 343

Tiran D (1995) Shiatsu. In: D Tiran, S Mack (eds) *Complementary Therapies for Pregnancy & Childbirth.* London: Bailliere Tindall

Elaine Cockburn
Sister Midwife
January 2002

Appendix 2

Useful bodies and training lists

The following is a list of professional bodies in various countries and regions that regulate shiatsu; they will be able to provide details of training courses in shiatsu and the regulations of the particular country.

Australia

Shiatsu Therapy Association of Australia (STAA), PO Box 598, Belgrave 3160, Victoria. Tel. (61) 03 9752 6711, www.staa.org.au

Canada

Shiatsu Therapy Association of British Columbia, PO Box 37005, 6495 Victoria Drive, Vancouver BC V5P 4W7. Tel. (1) 604 433 9495, www.shiatsutherapy.ca

Shiatsu Therapy Association of Ontario, 517, College Street, Suite 232, Toronto, Ontario M6G 4A2. Tel. (1) 416 923 7826, www.shiatsuassociation.com

Canadian Practitioners Association of Asian Medicine (CPAAM), 358, Dupont Street, Toronto. Tel. (1) 416 410 6419, www.cpaam.ca

Europe

The European Shiatsu Federation (made up of the national associations of nine member countries – Belgium, Germany, Spain, France, Ireland, Italy, Austria, Sweden and the UK). Website: www.shiatsu-esf.org

New Zealand

Shiatsu Association of Aotearoa (NZ) Inc., Box 238, Tauranga. Desiree Bailey (Treasurer), Tel. (64) (07) 5700188, email russ.b@xtra.co.nz

UK

Shiatsu Society, Eastlands Court, St Peters Road, Rugby, Warwickshire CV21 3AP. Tel. (44) (0) 1788 555 051, www.shiatsu.org

British Complementary Medicine Association, PO Box 5122, Bournemouth, BH8 0WG. Tel. (44) (0) 845 345 5977, www.bcma.co.uk

US

American Organisation for Bodywork Therapies of Asia (AOBTA), 1010, Haddonfield-Berlin Road, Suite 408, Voorhees, NJ 08043. Tel. (1) 856 782 1616, www.aobta.org

Worldwide

For details of specific courses on shiatsu in maternity care for midwives, shiatsu practitioners and massage therapists worldwide, contact Suzanne Yates at Well Mother, 24 Dunkerry Road, Windmill Hill, Bristol BS3 4LB, UK. Tel. (44) (0) 117 9632306, www.wellmother.org

Appendix 3

General questions relating to safety and diagnosis issues

Diagnosis for the non-shiatsu practitioner – how do I decide which technique to use and how will I know if it is the right one?

First of all, you can look up the condition/situation in the checklist and select a technique/meridian/point from here. What you work on will also depend on how much time you have. If you have less time, just work the points. If you have a little more time, you can work a whole meridian including the points. If you have even more time, or you are in a class situation, then you may want to give some of the exercises or visualizations for the meridians.

When you are working, you must pay attention to balancing the Kyo and Jitsu areas and get good feedback from the mother. If it feels right, continue. If unsure, discontinue and either try something else, or seek further advice from a practitioner or another midwife who has trained in shiatsu.

If there is a choice of techniques, you can consider:

- which meridian is most likely to be involved for this person – you can look up more information in the theory and practical chapters
- which area of the body seems the most Kyo and the most Jitsu and balance accordingly – you can do this by observing the mother's posture (remember, it is the Jitsu – tight, tense areas – that are the easiest to spot).

Can I make someone worse if I do the wrong thing?

As all energy is interconnected, it is quite difficult to work incorrectly provided you are responding to what you feel and getting good feedback from the mother. If you are doing the wrong thing it will feel wrong, both to you and to the mother. It is possible to go in too strongly or stay for too long, but both of these will feel wrong. If you stop as soon as you feel it is not right, then there will be no harm done. If you continue, you could make someone tired, you may make their energy unsettled, or you may aggravate underlying conditions. The worst you can do is aggravate an injury, but to do that you would have to work so that it felt uncomfortable at the time. Your best policy is feedback from the woman and checking your own discomfort.

Can I make myself worse by picking up on bad energy from other people?

It is difficult to do this if you apply the basic principles. The main thing to watch is if you are feeling tired or uncomfortable. If you are, then you need to find a way of changing your position so it is more comfortable. If you are tired, then you need to find a way of looking after your energy. See Chapter 8 to get some ideas about this.

Some people find it helpful to have a definite starting or ending point. It can be something like bringing your hands together, washing your hands or simply saying in your head, 'now I am beginning and connecting with the energy of another person', and, 'now I am finishing and letting the energy be in this other person's body'.

Are there any times/conditions when I should not use shiatsu?

I reiterate what I stated in Chapter 1. It is not possible to make a list of absolute contraindications, because the situations in which shiatsu is sometimes listed as contraindicated relate either to areas where shiatsu needs to be carried out alongside a Western approach – such as infection, inflammation, cancer, pre-eclampsia or thrombosis – or where knowledge of the relevant physiology will guide the correct use of shiatsu – such as not to work in a stimulating way on infections, and not to work directly over the area for thrombosis and varicose veins.

Index

Note: Numbers in bold refer to illustrations.